Khalid Krami
Benamara Ahmed
Radouani Mohammed

Road Infrastructures Faced with Climate Challenges

Khalid Krami
Benamara Ahmed
Radouani Mohammed

Road Infrastructures Faced with Climate Challenges

Geophysical Evaluation and Laboratory Testing: Case Studies in Morocco

ScienciaScripts

Road Infrastructures Faced with Climate Challenges

Geophysical Evaluation and Laboratory Testing: Case Studies in Morocco

Laboratory:

Mechanics, Mechatronics and Control Laboratory - L2MC

École Nationale Supérieure d'Arts et Métiers de Meknès.

Name of authors :

KRAMI Khalid

BENAMARA Ahmed

RADOUANI Mohammed

PREFACE

Managing road infrastructure is a major challenge for many countries, particularly in view of climatic conditions and increasing traffic loads. Morocco, with its vast road network, is no exception. Bituminous pavements, subjected to a wide range of mechanical and environmental stresses, are showing signs of deterioration that impact not only on road safety, but also on maintenance and rehabilitation costs.

This book is part of a research project aimed at improving our understanding of the mechanisms by which bituminous pavements deteriorate under the influence of climatic conditions and road traffic. By combining a geophysical approach, electrical resistivity tomography, and experimental laboratory tests, this work proposes concrete solutions for anticipating and preventing asphalt pavement damage.

The geophysical survey of four road sections in Morocco, before and during the winter season, sheds new light on the potential use of ERT as a preventive tool. In addition, laboratory evaluation of the water sensitivity and fracture toughness of asphalt mixes, particularly with the incorporation of hydrated lime, opens up interesting prospects for improving pavement durability.

This book is the fruit of several years of research and collaborative efforts between various players in the road sector. We hope it will contribute to enriching the technical knowledge of professionals, engineers and researchers, while providing practical recommendations for road infrastructure management in Morocco and elsewhere.

We would like to express our gratitude to all the people and institutions who have supported this research. Your contributions have been invaluable, helping to advance science in this crucial area.

SUMMARY

Asphalt pavements are subject to various environmental factors such as temperature changes, precipitation and traffic exposure, and can develop damage that compromises road safety and requires costly repairs. In order to gain a better understanding of these deterioration mechanisms, the first part of this book proposes the use of electrical resistivity tomography to assess the resistivity of the soil supporting road pavements. This analysis was carried out on four road sections, two on Route Régionale N°707 at Ifrane and two on Route Nationale N°13 at Azrou and Timhdit, before and during the winter season.

The results of this geophysical study will be invaluable in understanding the impact of winter conditions on pavement damage and crack formation in the wearing course. Electrical tomography will be used to create 2D images of soil resistivity, compared with asphalt cracking data obtained in the field. The images reveal a decrease in resistivity during winter, attributable to asphalt cracking, water infiltration and soil characteristics. This suggests that ERT could be used preventively to anticipate asphalt damage.

In the second part of the book, laboratory experiments were carried out to assess the water sensitivity and fracture resistance of asphalt mixes subjected to thermal cycling. Two types of aggregate were used, with hydrated lime incorporated as an additive. Samples were subjected to water resistance and semi-circular bending tests, SCB test, after being exposed to different thermal cycles simulating Moroccan climatic conditions.

The results showed that shale-based mixes were more sensitive to thermal cycling than limestone-based mixes, but the addition of hydrated lime improved the strength of both types of mix, especially the shale-based ones. The main aim of this research is to increase the durability of Moroccan roads while reducing maintenance costs.

CONTENTS

INTRODUCTION

Roads play an indispensable role in economic and social development, providing vital connectivity for communities and facilitating trade. However, asphalt pavements are subject to a multitude of stresses, from climatic variations to traffic pressures, exposing road users to potential risks and threatening road safety.

Management of the vast Moroccan road network, comprising some 26,360 km of roads[1]represents a major challenge for the Ministry of Equipment, Transport and Logistics. The considerable annual expenditure on pavement upkeep, rehabilitation and maintenance underscores the urgent need to find solutions to improve their durability while keeping costs under control. The continuous exposure of bituminous pavements to seasonal climatic variations and road traffic loads affects their strength, reducing their service life and ride quality.

In this context, this work aims to deepen our understanding of bituminous pavement deterioration mechanisms, by exploring two aspects: the impact of seasonal climatic variations and road traffic on pavement durability. To achieve this objective, we propose to use a non-destructive approach, the electrical tomography method. This method will enable us to map the electrical properties of pavement support soil, providing a detailed view of soil structure and its influence on pavement performance.

The aim of this work is also to assess the resistance to crack propagation in asphalt mixes, focusing specifically on the influence of aggregates and environmental conditions such as thermal stresses and humidity. To this end, we plan to use the semi-circular bending method, SCB test, on samples notched in mode I. This experimental approach will enable us to analyze the resistance of different asphalt mixes to mechanical and environmental stresses, taking particular account of the addition of hydrated lime as an additive, which can potentially improve pavement strength and durability.

By integrating these two research objectives, we can gain a better understanding of the factors influencing the durability of bituminous pavements, and it could help optimize road construction and maintenance practices, enabling more efficient use of financial resources and the promotion of more durable and resilient road infrastructure. This research work responds to the current concerns of managers in the sector, seeking to improve the quality and longevity of pavements, while ensuring the safety and fluidity of the Moroccan road network.

I. Materials used in asphalt mixes :

I.1 General information on asphalt :

I.1.1 Definition:

Asphalt mixes are materials composed mainly of aggregates (such as gravel, sand or aggregate) and bitumen. Bitumen is a viscous, hydrocarbon-based substance that acts as a binder, i.e. it binds aggregates together to form a solid, cohesive mass.

These asphalt mixes are widely used in the construction of roads, parking lots, airport runways and other transport infrastructures. They offer a smooth surface and must be durable and resistant to the stresses of road traffic and varying weather conditions.

Asphalt mixes can be classified into different categories according to their composition, gradation and properties, and can be used for different applications depending on the specific requirements of the construction project.

I.1.2 Bitumen:

Bitumen is a by-product of crude oil refining. The bitumen manufacturing process generally comprises two distinct stages: atmospheric distillation of crude oil, which initially produces a residual crude from the first refining tower, followed by distillation under reduced pressure, also known as vacuum distillation. This last stage recovers the bitumen from the bottom of the second refining tower. These bitumens are then subjected to various treatments, such as deasphalting, oxidation and blending, to produce bitumens with a variety of characteristics. Bitumens obtained directly by distillation are generally referred to as "bases" (hard and soft bases), and serve as raw materials for the manufacture of intermediate bitumens by blending. Among the range of bitumens frequently used in road construction, we distinguish [2]:

- ✓ Pure bitumens
- ✓ Hard grade bitumens
- ✓ Polymer-modified bitumens
- ✓ Multigrade bitumens

The two essential characteristics used in road engineering to differentiate bitumens are :

- ❖ The 25°C bitumen penetrability test is a method used to assess the consistency of bitumen at a specific temperature. During this test, a standard needle of precise size and weight is lowered vertically into a sample of bitumen heated to 25°C. Penetration is measured in millimeters after a certain time and with a certain load.
  More precisely, we measure the depth to which the standard needle penetrates vertically into the bitumen for 5 seconds under a standard load of 100 grams, in accordance with NM EN 1426[3]. This measurement gives an indication of the bitumen's hardness or consistency at this given temperature. The penetrability value can be used to classify different types of bitumen according to their consistency at 25°C, which is important in the design and formulation of bituminous mixes for various road applications.

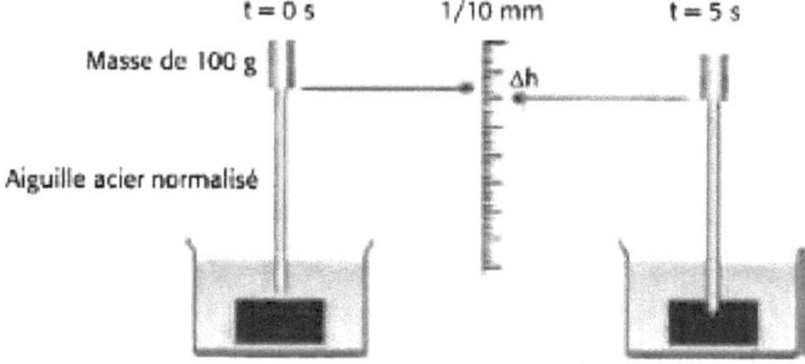

Figure 1Schematic diagram of the penetrability test.

❖ The ring-ball softening point test involves measuring the temperature at which the bitumen changes from its viscous state at 5°C to a more fluid state. For softening point values below 80°C, the test is carried out in a water bath; for values above 80°C, the test is carried out in a glycerine bath. This test is covered by standard NM EN 1427[4].

This test is important in the road industry as it provides an indication of the temperature at which bitumen becomes soft enough to lose its structural integrity, which can have an impact on the performance of bituminous pavements under different temperature conditions[2].

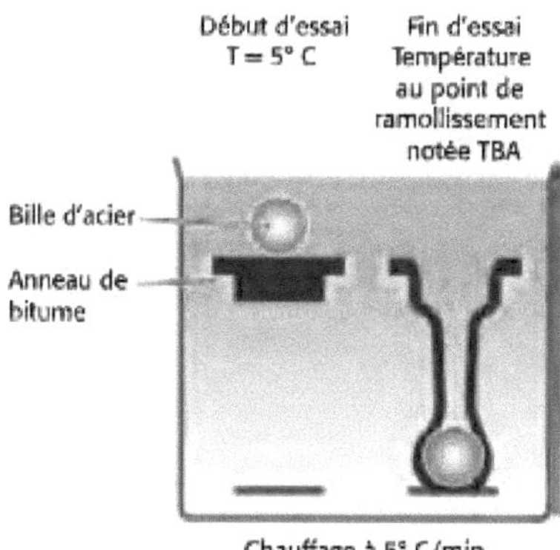

Figure 2Schematic diagram of the ball-ring temperature test.

I.1.3   Aggregates :

Aggregates refer to a variety of materials such as sand, gravel or crushed stone, ranging in size from 0 to 80 mm. These granular materials account for around 95% of the asphalt mix's total mass (constituting 80 to 85% of its volume).

The granularity of an aggregate mix is defined by the size of its components, which is crucial for its classification. Granular class is determined by quantifying the size of the smallest (d) and largest (D) grain in the mix.

The Moroccan guide to hot mix asphalt [5] defines the granular class as follows:

❖ An aggregate is classified as type d/D if it meets the following specifications:

> When the D/d ratio is greater than or equal to 2 :

✓ Rejection on sieve opening D is less than 10%,
✓ Passage over the opening sieve d is less than 10%,
✓ Passage over the d/2 sieve is less than 3%.

> When the D/d ratio is less than 2 :

✓ Rejection on sieve opening D is less than 15%,
✓ Passage over the opening sieve d is less than 15%,
✓ Passage over the d/2 sieve is less than 3%.

❖ For 0/D sand, the same definition is adopted for dimension D, with a rejection of less than 10%.

These criteria apply unless otherwise specified in the Cahier des Prescriptions Communes or the Cahier des Prescriptions Spéciales.

II. Impact of different types of stress on pavement structure degradation :

The asphalt mix must meet the requirements of road applications, where it is integrated into the pavement structure (see figure 3. This structure comprises: (i) the base course, which supports and transfers vehicle loads directly to the underlying soil, (ii) the wearing course, in direct contact with traffic and exposed to environmental conditions such as rain, snow, exposure to UV rays and heat, as well as the use of road de-icers during winter periods. The pavement body protects the subgrade against climatic variations. In this configuration, the pavement body is subjected to a complex combination of mechanical, thermal and physical-chemical stresses. All these external stresses eventually degrade the asphalt mix.

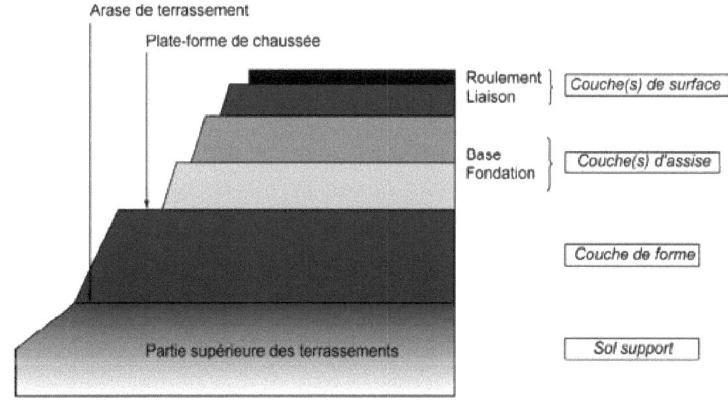

Figure 3Schematic representation of a pavement structure[6]

II.1 Mechanical stress :

The various pavement layers are subjected to compressive and tensile stresses due to the passage of traffic (see figure 4). Repeated traffic loads can lead to the formation of micro-cracks, which progressively progress and lead to the development of cracks through the material and then through the various pavement layers. In particular, surface cracking encourages water infiltration. These infiltrations can lead to a reduction in the soil's bearing capacity, the detachment of layers and thus accelerate material degradation[7].

Repeated loading of the pavement also leads to permanent deformations that can cause rutting of the road surface. These ruts can result from both deformation of the asphalt layers and differential settlement of the unbound layers beneath.

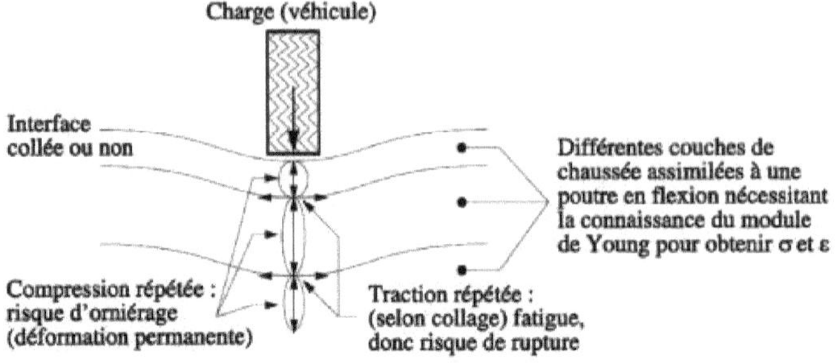

Figure 4Diagram of traffic-induced stresses[7]

II.2   Thermal loads :

Asphalt expands when exposed to high temperatures, and contracts when it gets colder. As a result, bituminous layers are particularly sensitive to the combined effects of traffic and temperature fluctuations. At higher temperatures, asphalt becomes relatively flexible and the risk of rutting increases under the impact of repeated vehicle loads. On the other hand, at lower temperatures, asphalt becomes brittle and the risk of thermal cracking increases.

In summary, three main temperature-related effects are observed on the behavior of asphalt mix: (i) aging of the material at elevated temperature, (ii) change in stiffness (complex modulus), and (iii) generation of stresses and strains within the material due to temperature variations resulting in thermal expansion and contraction.

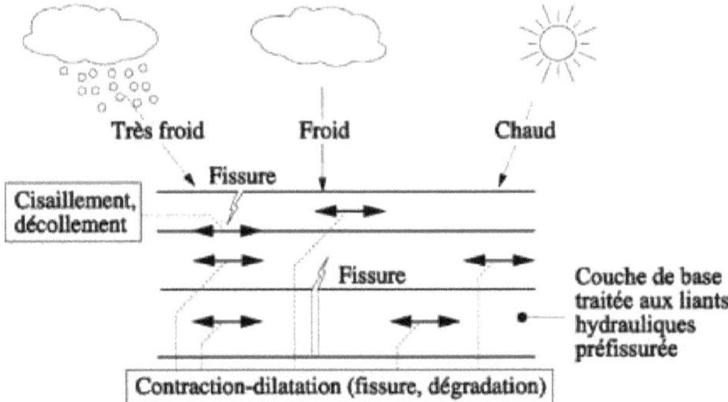

Figure 5Diagram of temperature-induced stresses in road structures[7]

II.3 Water solicitations :

Water damage is one of the most common causes of deterioration of pavement surface layers, as illustrated in figure 6. There are several ways in which water can enter the pavement. One possible route is infiltration through the surface layer, which can occur through microcracks, joints, material porosity, etc., fed by precipitation such as rain, snow or hail.

After each rainstorm, the material is exposed to water, which seeps through the binder/aggregate interface, weakening the asphalt and reducing its mechanical strength. The presence of water also accelerates damage caused by traffic. Several physico-chemical mechanisms are linked to the effect of water, including loss of adhesion and cohesion, pore pressure and water washout.

The loss of adhesion between binder and aggregate occurs progressively with the introduction of water, leading to the detachment and displacement of the binder. At the same time, the loss of cohesion of the bituminous mix is due to the reduced rigidity of the material caused by the penetration of water and the altered rheology of the binder, as illustrated in figure 7.

In addition, heat promotes water penetration into the asphalt by softening the material. Hydraulic pressure, combined with densification due to traffic, also accelerates the diffusion of water into the porous phase of the asphalt mix.

In addition, residual water trapped in the pavement several months after rainfall events can cause vapor pressure during summer periods. When this residual water freezes during cold periods, it increases in volume, leading to swelling and local cracking in the less compact and more fragile areas of the material.

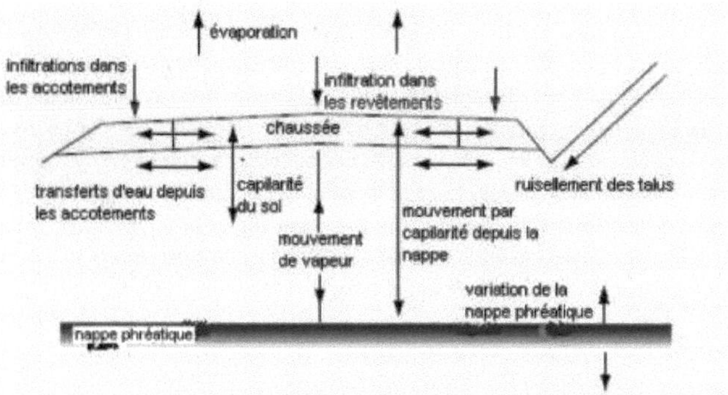

Figure 6:Water circulation in the subgrade and roadway

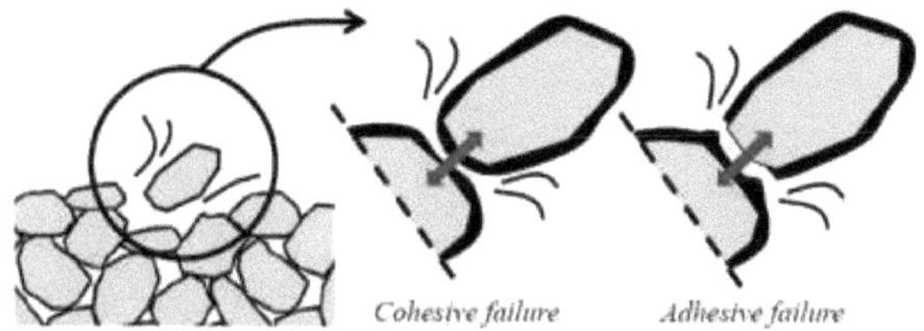

Figure 7:Asphalt delamination due to loss of adhesion and cohesion of components

II.4 Chemical stress :

In some regions with severe winter conditions, the use of road de-icers is essential to ensure road viability. These chemical substances lower the freezing point of water, making it easier to melt snow or ice even at sub-zero temperatures. Sodium chloride (NaCl) is widely used, accounting for around 99% of the tonnage spread.

During intense winter seasons, road managers have to resort to large quantities of salt to maintain acceptable traffic conditions for users. The use of salt on roads is regulated by specific standards that define its characteristics as a road melting agent.

In addition to sodium chloride, other fluxes such as calcium chloride (CaCl2) and magnesium chloride (MgCl2) are also used. These substances prevent the formation of ice at even lower temperatures than those reached with salt.

However, the application of these ice melters to the road surface not only causes the ice to melt, but also leads to thermal shock and osmotic pressure. These effects require careful management to minimize potential damage to roads and the environment.

In Morocco, road authorities in cold climatic zones, characterized by heavy snowfalls, also use pozzolan. This porous volcanic material offers an alternative to traditional chemical ice melters for snow and ice removal. Its absorbent properties enable it to soak up water from the surface, helping to reduce ice formation on roads by eliminating moisture.

In addition to its absorbent action, pozzolan can also improve vehicle traction when spread on snow-covered or icy roads. This improved traction reduces the risk of accidents by providing better grip for vehicle tires.

An added benefit of pozzolan is its environmentally-friendly nature. Unlike chemical ice melters such as salt, pozzolan is of natural origin and contains no harmful chemicals, making it a more environmentally-friendly option for road clearing.

However, it's important to note that the effectiveness of pozzolans can vary according to weather and temperature conditions. In some situations, it may be less effective than chemical ice melters in melting snow or ice. Its usefulness in snow removal operations in Morocco would depend on local climatic conditions and the availability of the material. A thorough evaluation of its effectiveness in these specific conditions would be necessary to determine its actual usefulness in snow removal operations in the country.

III.   Morocco's climate framework :

III.1 Brief description of Morocco's climate

Morocco's climate is highly diverse due to the country's varied geography, which includes coasts on the Atlantic Ocean and the Mediterranean Sea, mountains, plains and deserts. Overall, Morocco's climate can be described as Mediterranean on the coast, semi-arid inland and desert in the south, as illustrated in figure 8. Here is a brief description of each climatic region:

- ❖ Atlantic and Mediterranean coast :

On the Atlantic and Mediterranean coasts, the climate is Mediterranean, with hot, dry summers and mild, wet winters. Summer temperatures generally range from 25°C to 35°C, while winter temperatures remain mild, generally between 10°C and 20°C. Precipitation is more abundant during the winter months, but is generally moderate, generally between 300 and 500 mm per year, as illustrated in figure 9.

- ❖ Mountain regions :

The Rif, Atlas and Anti-Atlas mountains have a mountain climate, with temperatures dropping as altitude increases. The peaks can be snow-covered in winter. Precipitation is generally higher in mountainous regions, with variations depending on altitude and exposure, with annual precipitation ranging from 500 to 1000 mm, as illustrated in figure 9.

- ❖ Inner plain :

Morocco's interior plain has a semi-arid to arid climate. Summers are hot, with temperatures that can exceed 40°C, while winters are generally mild but can be cool, with temperatures sometimes dropping below 0°C at night. Precipitation is scarce in this region, and annual rainfall is relatively low, varying between 200 and 400 mm, as illustrated in figure 9.

- ❖ Sahara Desert:

In southern Morocco, the climate becomes desert-like. Temperatures can be extreme, often exceeding 45°C during the day and dropping considerably at night. Rainfall is very scarce, and water is a precious resource in this region. Sand winds can be frequent, especially during the hottest months.

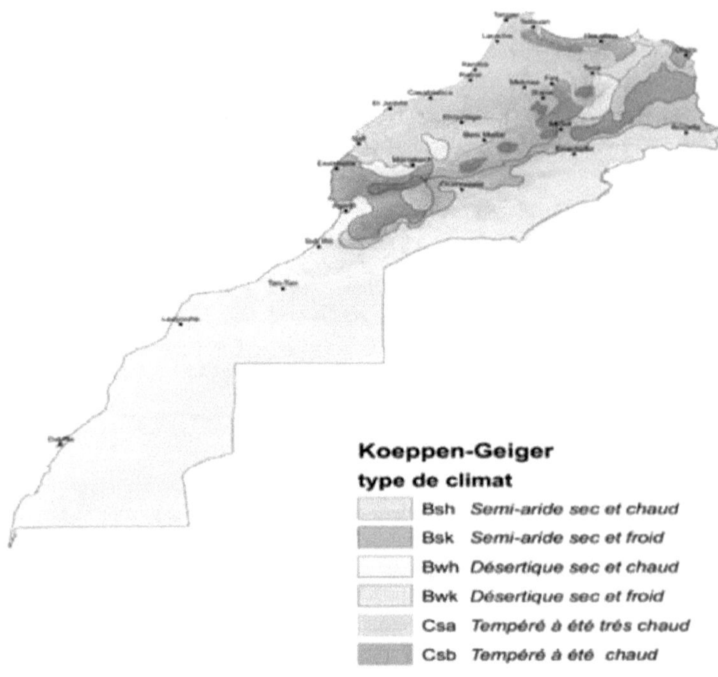

Figure 8Morocco's climate according to the Koeppen-Geiger index (1981-2010) [8]

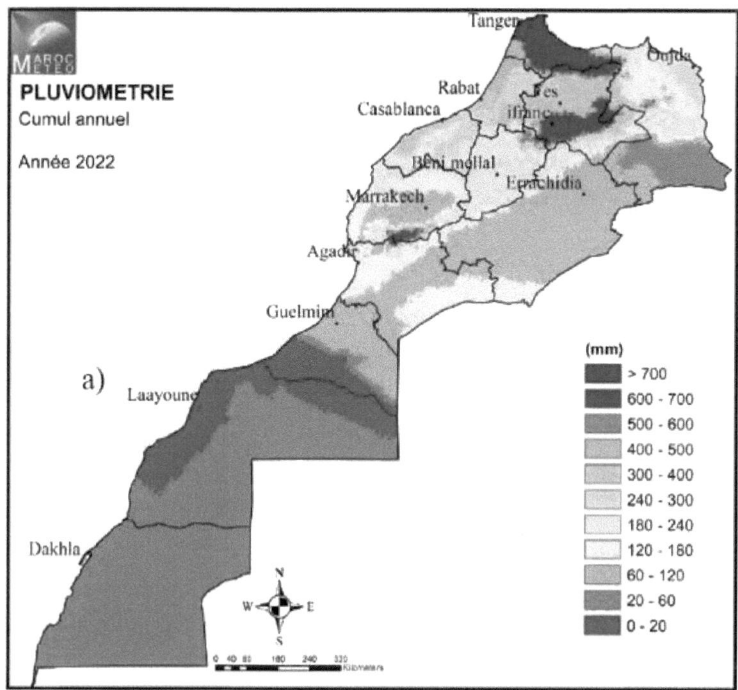

Figure 9Average annual rainfall map of Morocco[8]

III.2 Minimum temperature in Morocco:

A number of studies have attempted to describe Morocco's climate, both for the country as a whole and for specific areas. For example, in Midelt, a town in southeastern Morocco, monthly absolute minimum temperatures can be negative, ranging from -0.9 to -13.4°C in January and -0.8 to -13.5°C in December[9]. On average, monthly absolute minimum temperatures reach -4.7 and -3.6°C respectively for these two months, and around 80% of observations over several years indicate an absolute minimum temperature between -2 and -5°C[9].

In addition, the Direction de la Météorologie Nationale also provides a general description of the Moroccan climate, with historical data on the average temperature in selected Moroccan towns revealing that the coldest town in Morocco is Ifrane, with an average daily minimum temperature of -1°C over a 30-year period. Next come Errachidia, Ouarzazate and Bouarfa, with an average of 1°C during the coldest months of the year (December and January) [10].

A recent study by Lagrini et al.[11] was undertaken to map frost in Morocco. This study is based on the use of national meteorological data over a 30-year period, with the application of the following classification:

- ✓ Moderate frost: more than ten days with temperatures of -2°C or below.
- ✓ Frost-free: means no more than two days with temperatures of 0°C or below.
- ✓ Weak frost: a category including frost levels ranging from weak to severe.

17

The results of this study, presented in figure 10show that the weather stations for which data are available are classified as follows:

- ✓ Moderate frost: observed in Ifrane and Midelt.
- ✓ Weak frost: observed in Béni Mellal, Bouarfa, Meknès, Oujda and Ouarzazate.
- ✓ No frost: recorded in Tangier-Aéro, Larache, Rabat-Salé, Casa-Anfa, Al Hoceima, Nouasseur, Safi, Khouribga, Marrakech, Essaouira, Agadir-Massira, Sidi Ifni, Tan-Tan, Laâyoune and Dakhla.

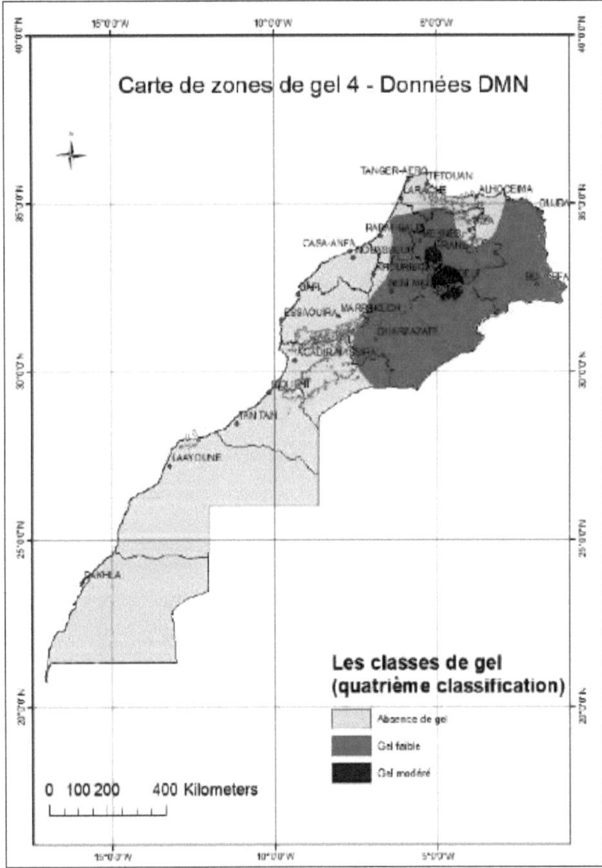

Figure 10:Frost map of Morocco according to the fourth classification - DMN data 1984-2014[11]

In addition, the same study also produced other spatial distribution maps based on the 30-year average (1984-2014) of the number of days per year when the daily minimum temperature is below -2°C and 0°C These maps were drawn up using data from the Direction de la Météorologie Nationale (DMN) from 26 weather stations, as illustrated in the following figures:

In figure 11the 30-year average of the number of days per year when the daily minimum temperature is below -2°C varies from 0 to 34. The highest values are recorded in Ifrane, with an average of over 30 days per year, followed by Midelt, with an average of over 10 days per year. The rest of the country shows values tending towards 0 for this indicator.

As for the figure 12shows the spatial distribution of the average number of days per year with daily minimum temperatures below 0°C. This average varies between 0 and 66, indicating the existence of areas in Morocco where frost persists for more than two months a year on average. The highest values are recorded in Ifrane, followed by Béni Mellal, Bouarfa, Midelt and Ouarzazate. In the north, west and south of the country, the number of days per year when the minimum temperature is negative tends towards 0, indicating that there is no risk of frost in these areas.

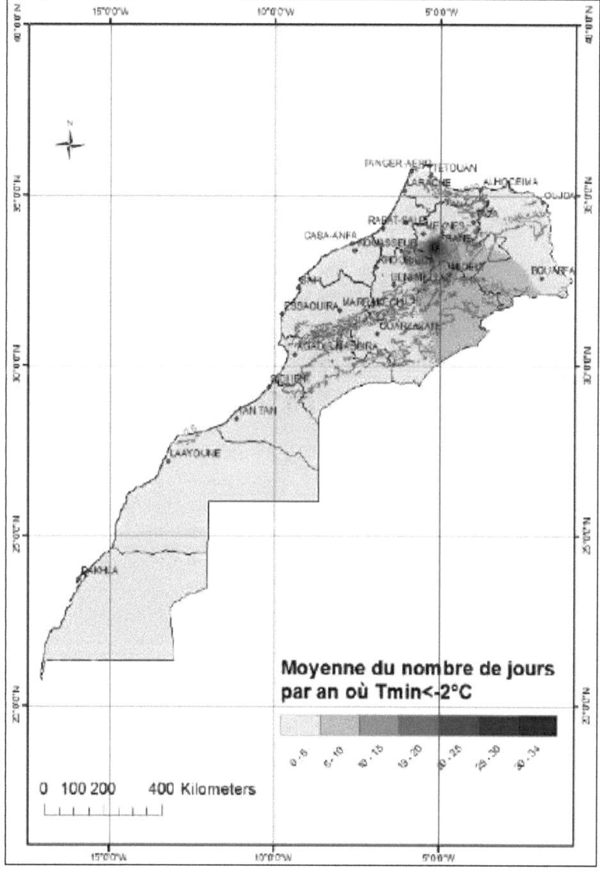

Figure 11:Annual average over 30 years of the number of days per year with daily minimum temperatures below -2°C in Morocco - DMN data 1984-2014[11]

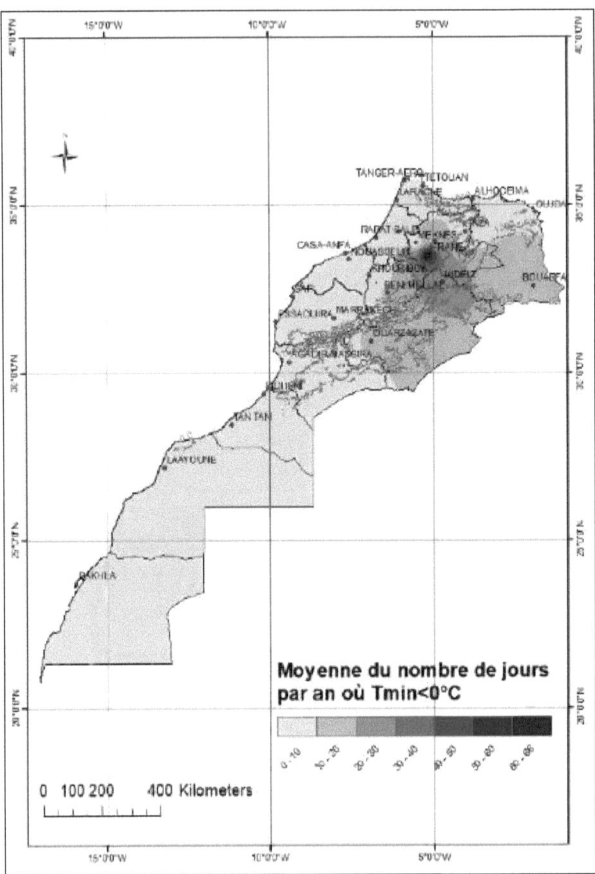

Figure 12:Annual average over 30 years of the number of days per year with daily minimum temperatures below -2°C in Morocco - DMN data 1984-2014[11]

III.3 Maximum temperature in Morocco :

A number of studies have been carried out to describe Morocco's climate, both for the country as a whole and for specific areas. For example, according to a study by Ionesco and colleagues [12]average maximum temperatures in the hottest month, usually July, exceed 30°C throughout the country, with the exception of the Atlantic coast and high mountain regions.

Rhanem [9] noted that in the town of Midelt, July and August 1988 recorded the highest average daily maximum temperatures, at 32.6°C and 32.1°C respectively. The values recorded each year vary between 30.3°C and 34.2°C for July, and between 30.4°C and 34.2°C for August. During the day, temperatures often reach 35 to 36°C in July, while the range is wider in August, from under 34°C to over 37°C. He also noted that the number of days with temperatures above 30°C varies from 36 to 87 per year, with an average of 67.6. Temperatures in excess of 30°C can be observed from May to September, with a particularly high frequency in July and August, months in which daily maximum temperatures rarely fall below this value.

According to historical meteorological data available on the website of the National Meteorological Directorate, the hottest cities in Morocco are Beni Mellal, Bouarfa, Kasba Tadla, Marrakech, Ouarzazate and Errachidia, with maximum daily temperatures ranging from 35°C to 39°C, calculated over an annual average of more than 30 years. [10].

A recent study by Lagrini et al.[11] was undertaken to map maximum temperatures in Morocco. This study is based on the use of national meteorological data over a 30-year period, with the application of the following classification:

- ✓ High maximum temperature: More than 10 days per year with a daily maximum temperature above 38°C
- ✓ Low maximum temperature: Less than 2 days per year with a daily maximum temperature above 35°C
- ✓ Moderate maximum temperature: Between the two

The results of this study, presented in figure 13show that the weather stations for which data are available are classified as follows:

- ✓ High maximum temperature: Béni Mellal, Bouarfa, Khouribga, Marrakech, Meknes, Ouarzazate, Sale, Taza.
- ✓ Moderate maximum temperature: Tanger Aero, Tétouan, Oujda, Larache, Rabat, Casa-Anfa, Nouasseur, Safi, Agadir Massira, Sidi Ifni, Tan-Tan, Lâayoune
- ✓ Low maximum temperature: Al Hoceima, Dakhla, Essaouira, Ifrane, Midelt.

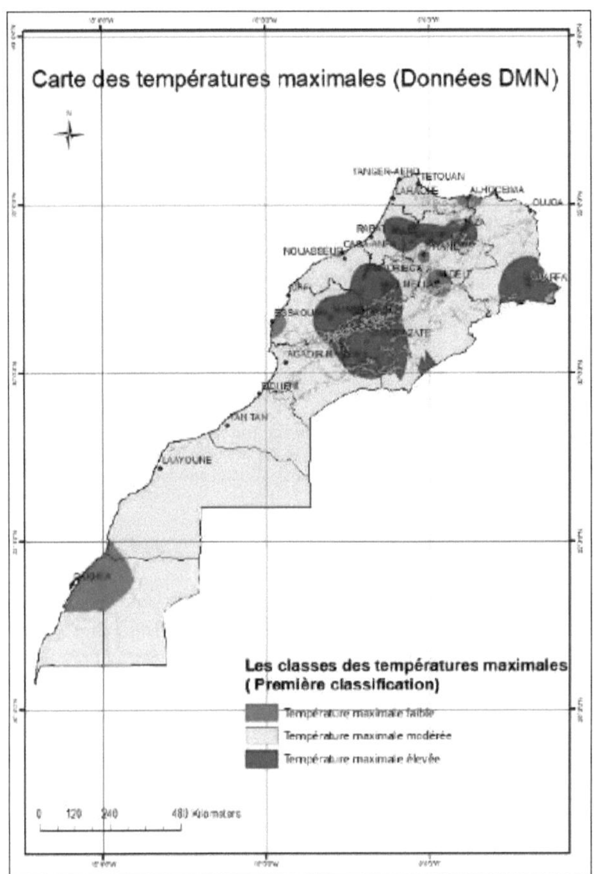

Figure 13 Map of maximum temperatures in Morocco according to the first classification - DMN data 1984-2014[11]

In addition, the same study also generated other spatial distribution maps, based on the 30-year average (1984-2014), of the number of days per year when the daily maximum temperature exceeds 38°C and 35°C. These maps were developed using data from the Direction de la Météorologie Nationale (DMN) from 26 weather stations, as illustrated in the following figures:

The figure 14 shows that the 30-year average of the number of days per year when the maximum daily temperature exceeds 38°C varies between 0 and 35 days. The highest values are recorded in Béni Mellal, Marrakech and Ouarzazate, with an average between 30 and 35 days per year, followed by Bouarfa and Taza, with an average between 25 and 30 days. The figure also shows that Rabat Salé averages between 15 and 20 days a year when the maximum temperature exceeds 38°C.

As for the figure 15shows that most areas in Morocco are characterized by an average of between 20 and 50 days per year when the maximum temperature exceeds 35°C. However, higher values are observed in the provinces of Ouarzazate, Marrakech, Béni Mellal and Bouarfa. However, higher values are observed in the provinces of Ouarzazate, Marrakech, Béni Mellal and Bouarfa. On the other hand, some areas, mainly on the coast, such as Tétouan, Tangier, Essaouira, Tan-Tan and Dakhla, have very low average temperatures, ranging from 0 to 10 days a year.

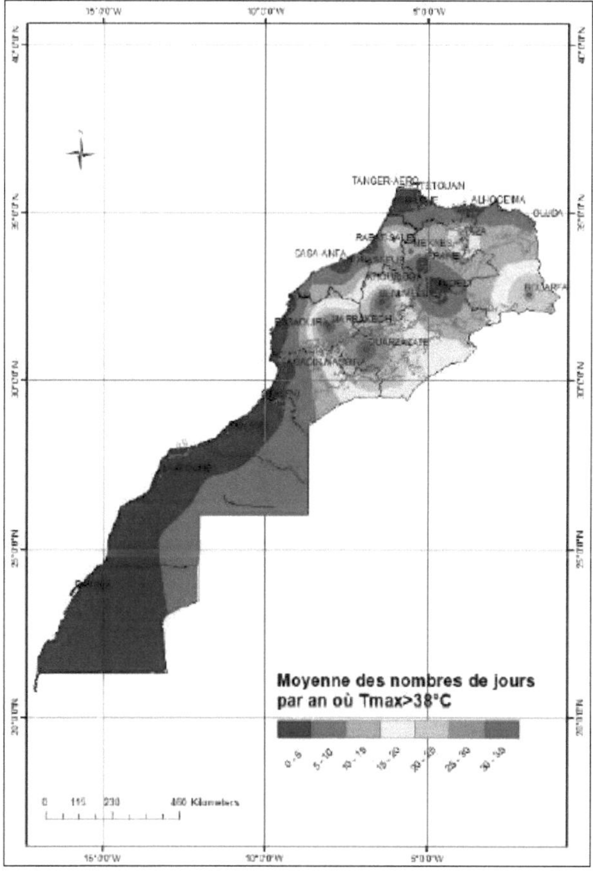

Figure 14:Annual average over 30 years of the number of days per year with daily maximum temperatures above 38°C in Morocco - DMN data 1984-2014[11]

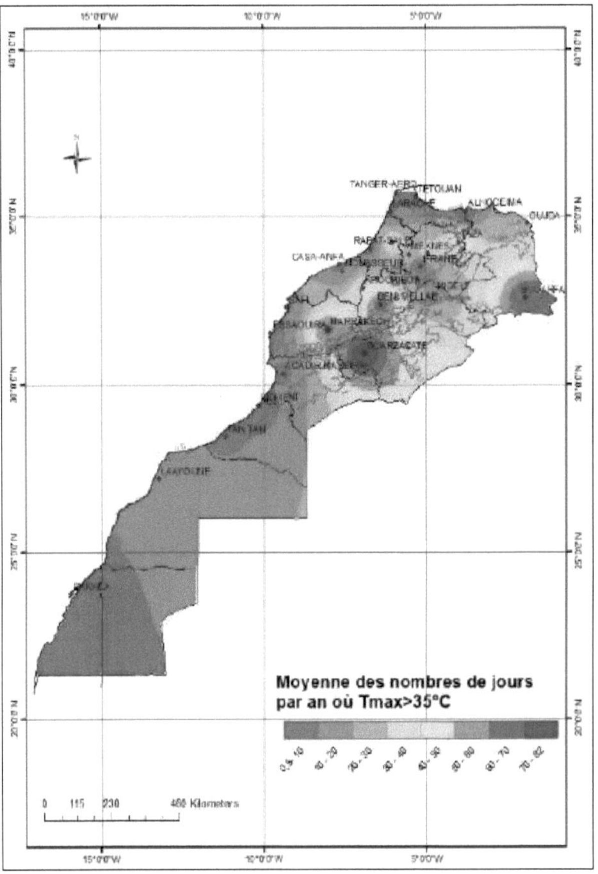

Figure 15:Annual average over 30 years of the number of days per year with daily maximum temperatures above 35°C in Morocco - DMN data 1984-2014[11]

III.4 Thermal gradient in Morocco :

III.4.1 Thermal gradient according to DMN data :

Historical meteorological data reveal that the cities with the highest temperature ranges in Morocco are : Ouarzazate, Beni Mellal, Marrakech and Kasbat Tadla, with an average varying between 18°C and 20°C throughout the year, while Bouarfa, Fes-Sais, Ifrane, Khouribga, Errachidia, Sidi Slimane and Taza follow closely behind with average amplitudes between 15 and 18°C [10]. These figures represent averages, implying that daily temperature variations

24

can be much greater in some cases, particularly in areas far from urban centers and mountain ranges.

A recent study by Lagrini et al.[11] was undertaken to map the thermal gradient of Morocco. This study is based on the use of national meteorological data over a 30-year period, with the application of the following classification:

- ✓ High thermal gradient: daily thermal gradient above 20°C for at least 10 days a year
- ✓ Low thermal gradient: Daily thermal gradient above 15°C for 2 days or less
- ✓ Moderate thermal gradient: Between the two categories.

The results of this study, presented in figure 16show that the weather stations for which data are available are classified as follows:

- ✓ High thermal gradient: Béni Mellal, Meknes, Nouasseur, Oujda and Rabat-Salé.
- ✓ Low thermal gradient: Essaouira.
- ✓ Moderate thermal gradient : All the rest of the Kingdom.

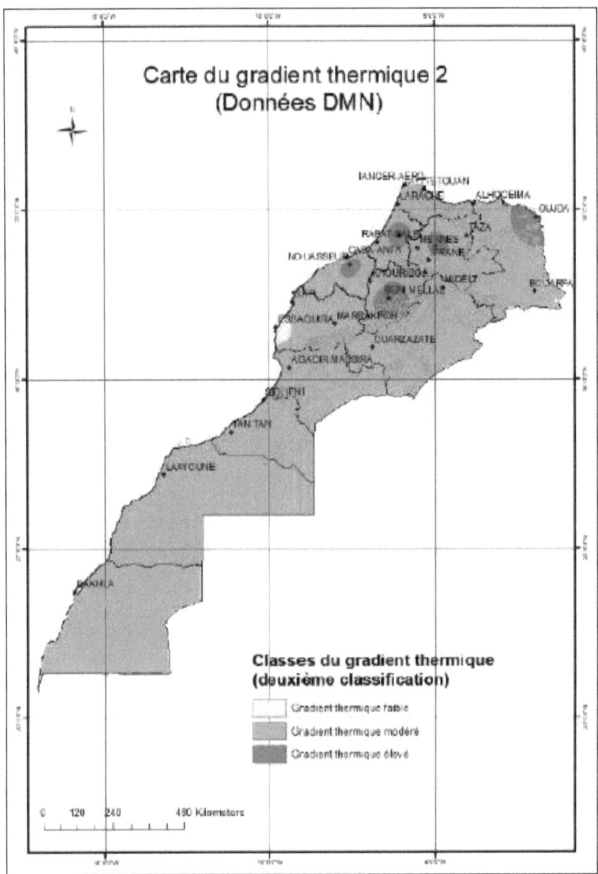

Figure 16Thermal gradient map of Morocco according to the first classification - DMN data 1984-2014. [11]

In addition, the same study also generated another spatial distribution map, based on the 30-year average (1984-2014), the distribution of the number of days per year when the daily thermal gradient is greater than 20°C. This map was drawn up using data from the Direction de la Météorologie Nationale (DMN) from 26 weather stations, as illustrated in figure 17.

The figure 17 illustrates the spatial distribution of the number of days per year when the daily temperature gradient exceeds 20°C. In this context, the averages show significant values, ranging from 0 to 62 days. The highest values are found near the Beni Mellal weather station, followed by Ouarzazate, Marrakech, Rabat-Salé, Ifrane and Oujda.

The results show that, for the southern regions of the country, the average number of days when the thermal gradient exceeds 20°C is very low, ranging from 0 to 10 days. However, these regions are known to be characterized by a climate that is very hot during the day and very cold at night, a variation that is not reflected in the map obtained. This lack of representation is due to the fact that the weather stations available in southern Morocco are all located along the coast, which makes their climate significantly different from that of areas further away from the coast.

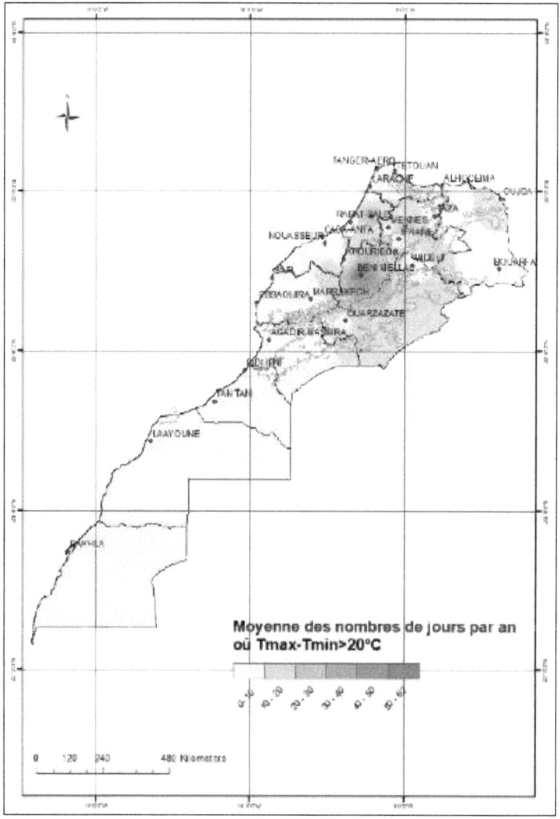

Figure 17:Annual average over 30 years of the number of days per year when the daily thermal gradient is greater than 20°C in Morocco - DMN data 1984-2014[11]

III.4.2   Thermal gradient according to CFSR data :

A recent study by Lagrini et al.[11]   was undertaken to map the thermal gradient of Morocco. This study relies on the use of data based on the re-analysis of the climate prediction system (CFSR), completed over a 36-year period from 1979 to 2014, with the application of the following classification:

- ✓ High thermal gradient: daily thermal gradient above 25°C for at least 10 days a year
- ✓ Low thermal gradient: Daily thermal gradient above 20°C for 2 days or less
- ✓ Moderate thermal gradient: Between the two categories.

The results of this study, presented in figure 18show that using thirty-year averages of maximum and minimum temperatures for 927 points in the CFSR database, we find the following:

✓ High thermal gradient: Areas located in the provinces of Azilal, Béni Mellal, Midelt, Figuig, Rhamna, Youssoufia, Assa Zag, Tan-Tan, Tarfaya, Laâyoune, Es-Semara, Oued Ed Dahab and Aouesserd.
✓ Low thermal gradient: Errachidia, Zagora, Tata, Tiznit, Sidi Ifni, Chtouka Ait Baha, Agadir Ida-Outanane, Sidi Bennour, Safi, Salé, El Hajeb , Khémissat, Ifrane, Boulemane, Kenitra, Larache, Tétouan, Tanger-Assilah, Fahs Anjra.
✓ Moderate thermal gradient: The rest of the country represents more than 50% of the Kingdom's surface area.

This map gives a more accurate characterization of the thermal gradient, especially for southern areas, given the good distribution of points where data are available. This map is therefore considered to be the thermal gradient map produced using CFSR data.

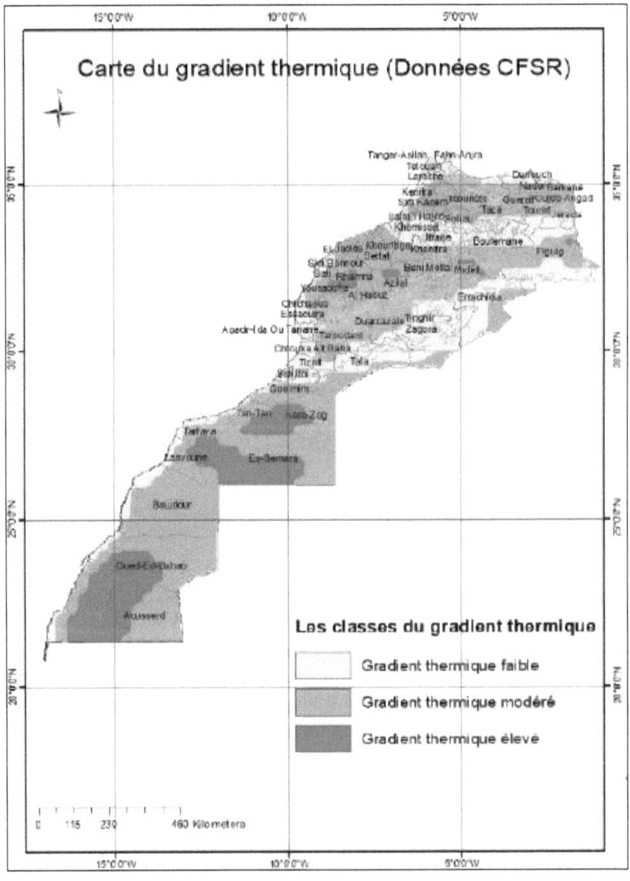

Figure 18Map of Morocco's thermal gradient according to the first classification - CFSR data[11]

In addition, the same study also generated another spatial distribution map, using CFSR data, the distribution of the number of days per year when the daily thermal gradient is greater than 20°C, as illustrated in the following figure :

The figure 19 shows the spatial distribution of the 30-year average number of days per year when the difference between daily maximum and daily minimum temperatures exceeds 20°C in Morocco. The results show that this average varies between 0 and 160 days per year across the country.

The highest values are found in the extreme south-west of the country, far from the coast, precisely in parts of the provinces of Oued Ed-Dahab and Aousserd, where they range between 120 and 160 days a year. The rest of these two provinces, as well as areas to the south of Es-Smara province, have relatively high values of between 80 and 120 days a year.

Values between 40 and 80 days a year are found in the provinces of Boulemane, Midelt, Fqih Ben Saleh, Kelâat Es-Sraghna, Settat, Rehamna, Khouribga, Marrakech, Youssoufia, Beni Mellal, Taounate, Taza, Guercif, Assa Zag and parts of Tarfaya, Tan Tan, Es-Semara and Figuig. The rest of the country is characterized by relatively low values, ranging from 0 to 40 days per year.

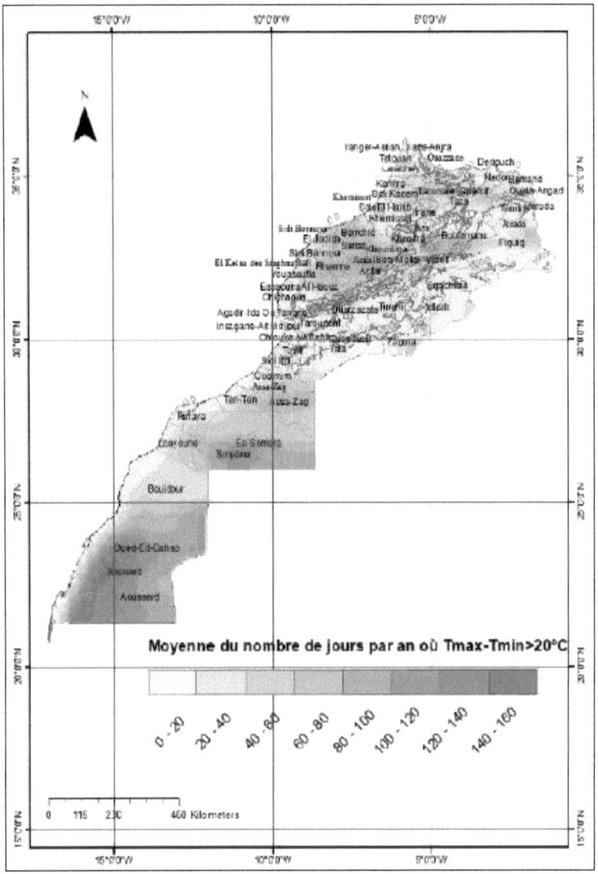

Figure 19:Annual average over 30 years of the number of days per year when the daily thermal gradient is greater than 20°C in Morocco - CFSR data 1984-2014[11]

IV.   Method used to design asphalt pavements with respect to climatic conditions:

IV.1 Principle of the sizing process :

Among the methods for designing bituminous pavements in Morocco, standard NF P 98-086 version 2019[13] is applied. This standard proposes both a mechanical approach and a consideration of frost in the design of the structure. Mechanical dimensioning aims to ensure that the chosen structure is capable of withstanding the cumulative traffic of heavy goods vehicles over the defined service life. This involves comparing the stresses and strains calculated using a linear elastic model with admissible values determined on the basis of the strength of materials under repeated loads, taking into account various adjustment coefficients for design reliability and rigid pavement discontinuities. Calculated stresses in the pavement must be less than or equal to permissible values. The minimum layer thickness is determined by successive iterations in order to meet this criterion.

Next, the structure resulting from the mechanical calculation is subjected to a freeze/thaw check. This involves calculating the permissible frost index for the pavement, which must be higher than the winter reference frost index. This step may entail adjustments to the thicknesses determined by the mechanical calculation. If the increase in thickness is not sufficient to dimension the pavement structure, it may be necessary to modify the pavement or soil materials, or even the subgrade. It is important to emphasize that this step is not implemented in Morocco, due to the lack of studies defining the permissible frost index for the pavement and the winter reference frost index in the Moroccan context.

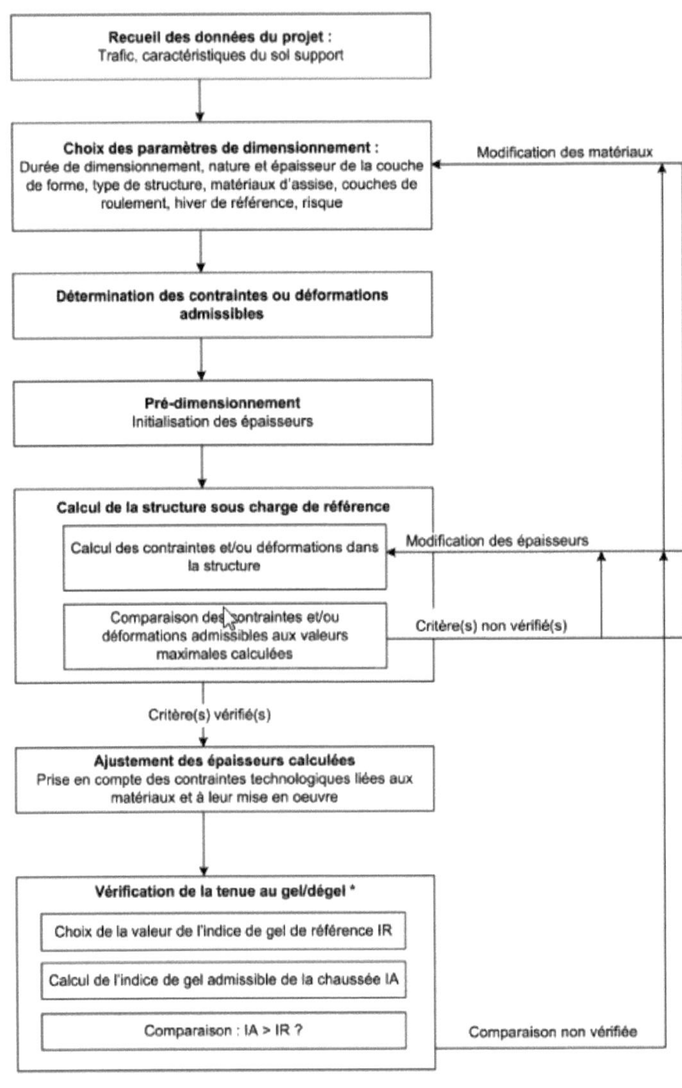

Figure 20Schematic diagram of the sizing method for new road pavements[13].

IV.2 Mechanical sizing :

The mechanical dimensioning of the structure is based on several aspects[13] :

- ❖ Assessment of heavy goods vehicle traffic in the project in terms of loading cycles, represented by a number of NE cycles for a reference axle (single axle with twin wheels and a total load of 130 kN according to standard NF P 98-082).
- ❖ Calculation of permissible stresses, taking into account the value of NE, the risk of permanent deformation of the subgrade and unbound layers, and the risk of fatigue of bound layers (bituminous or hydraulic).
- ❖ Calculation of the stresses exerted on the structure by the reference load (twin-wheeled half-axle loaded to 65 kN as per standard NF P 98-082), using a multi-layer, homogeneous and isotropic linear elastic model (Burmister model) in which the stiffness of the materials is described by a Young's modulus and a Poisson's ratio. The soil and any subgrade are represented by a semi-infinite layer with a Young's modulus corresponding to that of the subgrade class in question.
- ❖ The choice of a load frequency or load duration, as well as an equivalent temperature for bituminous materials, to determine the material properties to be used in the dimensioning method. In general, a load frequency of 10 Hz and a load duration of 0.02 s are adopted. The equivalent temperature (θeq) is defined as the constant temperature that would cause the same annual cumulative damage to the structure as that caused by actual temperature variations over the year.

In Morocco, pavement dimensioning is carried out using equivalent temperatures generally set between 19 and 25°C by the responsible authorities. For example, the Ministry of Equipment, Transport, Logistics and Water generally opts for a value of 25°C, while the Société Nationale des Autoroutes du Maroc favors 19°C. To our knowledge, these values are not supported by any prior study and appear to be based solely on the initial administrative decision [14].

IV.2.1 Converting traffic into equivalent axles :

Heavy goods vehicle traffic expected to use the roadway during its design life, expressed as the cumulative number of heavy goods vehicles NPL, is converted into an equivalent number NE of reference axle passes (NF P 98-082).

For mechanical pavement design, it is also necessary to determine the cumulative traffic over the design period.

The mechanical design of the pavement is carried out by considering the cumulative heavy goods vehicle traffic for the selected design period, represented by the Cumulative Number of Heavy Goods Vehicles (*NPL*) and calculated as followsEquation 1 .

Equation 1 calculation of NPL.

$$NPL = 365 \times TMJA \times C$$

Where:

- ✓ *NPL* is the cumulative number of heavy goods vehicles;
- ✓ *AADT* is the Average Annual Daily Traffic, expressed as the number of HGVs/day/direction for the busiest lane in the year of commissioning or the period under consideration;
- ✓ *This* is the cumulative traffic factor for the design period.

Calculation of the C coefficient depends on the assumption of growth in heavy goods vehicle traffic. Its expression for a cumulative period of n years is given in Equation 2 for arithmetic growth, and inEquation 3 for geometric growth.

Equation 2:calculating C for arithmetic growth

$$C = n \times \left(1 + \frac{(n-1) \times \tau}{2}\right)$$

Where:

- ✓ τ is the arithmetic growth rate of heavy goods vehicle traffic in % ;
- ✓ n is the cumulative period in years.

Equation 3:calculating C for geometric growth

$$C = \frac{(1+\tau)^n - 1}{\tau}$$

Where:

- ✓ τ is the geometric growth rate of heavy goods vehicle traffic in % ;
- ✓ n is the cumulative period in years.

For dimensioning purposes, the number of heavy goods vehicles accumulated over the dimensioning period (NPL) is converted into a reference Equivalent Number of Axles (NE) using the average aggressiveness coefficient for CAM traffic, as shown inEquation 4.

Equation 4Calculation of NE as a function of NPL

$$NE = NPL \times CAM$$

Where:

- ✓ NE is the equivalent number of reference axles;
- ✓ NPL is the number of trucks calculated for the dimensioning period d ;
- ✓ CAM is the average aggressiveness coefficient for the traffic defined

IV.2.2 Average aggressiveness coefficient (CAM) values :

Standard NF P 98-086 version 2019 recommends the use of calculation values for the average aggressivity coefficient (CAM) specific to different pavement types, as shown in Table 1and Table 2 and Table 3are used.

Table 1Average Aggressivity Coefficients as a function of traffic and type of material for motorway pavements[13]

	T2	T1	T0	TS	Tex
CAM Matériaux Bitumineux			0,8		
CAM Matériaux Traités aux Liants Hydrauliques et béton			1,3		
CAM Sol, GNT			1		

Table 2Average Aggressivity Coefficients as a function of traffic and type of material for non-motorway pavements[13]

	T5	T4	T3-	T3+	T2, T1, T0
CAM Matériaux Bitumineux	0,3	0,3	0,4	0,5	0,5
CAM Matériaux Traités aux Liants Hydrauliques et béton	0,4	0,5	0,6	0,6	0,8
CAM Sol, GNT	0,4	0,5	0,6	0,75	1

Table 3Average Aggressivity Coefficients as a Function of Traffic and Material Type for Urban Pavements [13]

	Voie de desserte	Voie de distribution	Voie principale à trafic lourd
CAM Matériaux Bitumineux	0,1	0,2	0,2
CAM Matériaux Traités aux Liants Hydrauliques et béton	0,1	0,2	0,4
CAM sur giratoire	0,2	0,5	1,0

IV.2.3 Calculation of permissible loads:

The dimensioning method considers two damage mechanisms, each associated with a distinct expression of permissible stresses:

- ✓ Fatigue damage to bituminous materials is taken into account through their maximum permissible reversible horizontal extensional deformation εt adm.
- ✓ Damage due to the accumulation of permanent deformations in untreated materials is taken into account through their maximum permissible reversible vertical deformation εz,adm.

IV.2.3.1 Permissible deformation criterion for bituminous materials, εt adm :

For a bituminous layer subjected to extensional stress due to bending, the permissible deformation for the equivalent temperature θeq is calculated according toEquation 5.

Equation 5Permissible deformation equation for bituminous materials

$$\varepsilon_{t,adm} = \varepsilon_6(10\ ^{\circ}\text{C} : 25\ \text{Hz}) \times \sqrt{\frac{E(10\ ^{\circ}\text{C} : 10\ \text{Hz})}{E(\theta_{eq} : 10\ \text{Hz})}} \times \left(\frac{NE}{10^6}\right)^b \times k_c \times k_r \times k_s$$

Where:

- ✓ ε6(10 °C; 25 Hz) is the parameter of the bituminous material's fatigue law, representing the deformation leading to a service life of 106 cycles. ε6 is determined by the standardized two-point bending fatigue test (NF EN 12697-24, Annex A). This test is performed at 10°C and 25 Hz;
- ✓ b is the slope of the fatigue law for bituminous material $(-1 < b < 0)$;
- ✓ E (10 °C; 10 Hz) is the modulus of rigidity at 10 °C and 10 Hz , obtained in accordance with standard NF EN 12697-26, :
- ✓ E (θeq; 10 Hz) is the modulus of rigidity at θeq and 10 Hz , obtained in accordance with standard NF EN 12697-26 ;
- ✓ NE is the number of passes of the reference axle;
- ✓ kc, kr, ks are the adjustment coefficients.

IV.2.3.1.1 Adjustment coefficients :

Various coefficients, kr, ks and kc, are used to adjust the value of the permissible deformation in the fatigue cracking criterion for layers treated with bituminous binders. These coefficients are defined in the following paragraphs.

- ❖ **Risk coefficient kr** :

Using the risk coefficient r, the design method incorporates a probabilistic approach to pavement service life, taking into account possible variations in the mechanical properties of materials and pavement layer thicknesses.

The risk represents, for the design period, the expectation (according to probability theory) of the linear proportion of pavement to be rebuilt in the absence of any structural maintenance work during this period.

The risk coefficient is calculated according toEquation 6 as follows

Equation 6:calculation of risk coefficient kr

$$k_r = 10^{-u \times b \times \delta} \quad \text{et} \quad \delta = \sqrt{S_N{}^2 + \left(\frac{c \times S_h}{b}\right)^2}$$

With :

- ✓ u is the value of the random variable of the reduced centered normal distribution associated with the risk r. defined in standard 98-086 version 2019 ;
- ✓ b is the slope of the fatigue line for the layer material under consideration, the values of which, for each
- ✓ material class, are defined in standard 98-086 version 2019 $(-1 < b < 0)$;
- ✓ SN is the standard deviation on the decimal logarithm of the number of cycles leading to fatigue failure, whose values for each material class are defined in standard 98-086 version 2019;
- ✓ Sh is the standard deviation of the thickness of the layers of materials used, expressed in meters. The values for each class of material are defined in standard 98-086 version 2019;

✓ *c* is the coefficient associating the variation in deformation with the variation in pavement thickness, expressed in m-1. The value of *c* determined from the study of standard structures is equal to 2 m-1.

❖ *Platform coefficient ks :*

The ks coefficient takes into account any variations in the bearing capacity of the supporting platform, which are all the more detrimental to the structure when the bearing capacity of the platform is low. This coefficient affects only the layer resting on the platform and depends on the bearing capacity of the latter, as defined in Table 4:

Table 4ks values taken into account as a function of the bearing capacity of the platform or the modulus of the layer underlying the layer of bonded material under consideration[13]

Module	E < 50 MPa	50 MPa ≤ E < 80 MPa	80 MPa ≤ E < 120 MPa	E ≥ 120 MPa
k_s	1/1,2	1/1,1	1/1,065	1

❖ *Calibration coefficient* kc

The calibration coefficient, noted *kc*, corrects the discrepancy between the predictions of the calculation approach and the observed behavior of real pavements.

IV.2.3.2 Permissible deformation criterion for untreated materials and pavement-bearing soils, εz,adm :

For a layer of untreated material and for the soil, the permissible stress is the vertical deformation at the surface of the layer, calculated according toEquation 7.

Equation 7Permissible deformation equation for untreated materials and pavement-bearing soils

$$\varepsilon_{z,adm} = A \times (NE)^b$$

Where:

✓ *A, b* are parameters dependent on traffic level, type of material and structure, defined in standard 98-086 version 2019 (- 1 < *b* < 0);
✓ *NE* is the number of passes of the reference axle.

IV.2.4 Determination of loads induced in the structure by the reference load :

Calculations of the stresses induced in the pavement structure under the reference load are carried out using a multi-layer semi-infinite linear elastic model (Burmister model). This model represents the entire pavement structure as a series of layers, with constant thicknesses in plan. Only the lower layer, whose upper limit corresponds to the subgrade, is infinite in depth. Each layer consists of a homogeneous, isotropic material with linear elastic behavior characterized by a Young's modulus (E) and a Poisson's ratio (v). Conditions at the interfaces can be either bonded or sliding, depending on the materials in contact. The semi-bonded interface assumption is used, defined as the average of the results obtained with a bonded interface and a sliding interface in succession.

The values of the mechanical parameters (E, v) to be taken into account, as well as the conditions at the interfaces, depend on the specific nature of the materials, and are provided in standard NF P 98-086.

The calculation is carried out for the reference load corresponding to a 65 kN twin-wheel half-axle. It is represented by two discs with a radius of 0.125 m, their centers spaced 0.375 m apart, and applying a uniform pavement surface pressure of 0.662 MPa. The loads (reversible stresses and strains) are calculated at the base of the bonded layers and at the top of the unbonded layers, as shown in Figure 21.

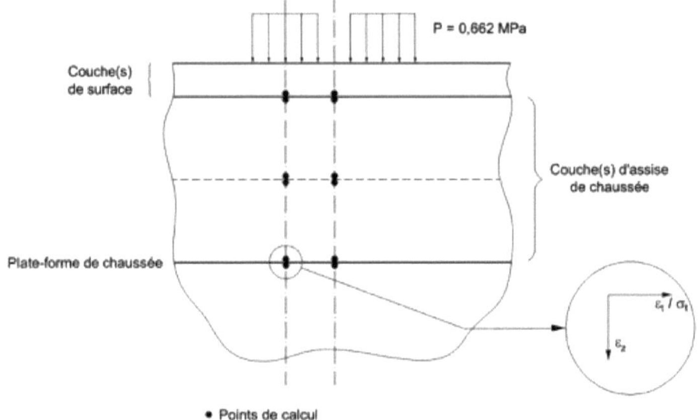

Figure 21 Reference load and calculation point[13]

IV.2.4.1 Design characteristics of pavement materials :

IV.2.4.1.1 Untreated gravel :

The mechanical parameters of untreated gravel to be taken into account when dimensioning structures vary according to their classification into categories, the type of structure and whether they are used as a base course or sub-base.

The Table 5 provides modulus of rigidity values for untreated gravel used in pavement design. Poisson's ratio is set at 0.35 for these materials.

Chaussées pour lesquelles la classe de trafic est inférieure ou égale à T3	
Catégories définies dans la norme NF EN 13285	
couche de base	catégorie 1 : E_{GNT} = 600 MPa
	catégorie 2 : E_{GNT} = 400 MPa
	catégorie 3 : E_{GNT} = 200 MPa
couche de fondation *(GNT subdivisée en sous-couches de 0,25 m d'épaisseur indicée par i croissant de bas en haut)*	E_{GNT} {1} = 3 $E_{plateforme-support}$ E_{GNT} {sous-couche i} = k E_{GNT} {sous-couche (i-1)} k variant selon la catégorie de la GNT <table><tr><td>Catégorie</td><td>1</td><td>2</td><td>3</td></tr><tr><td>k</td><td>3</td><td>2,5</td><td>2</td></tr></table> E_{GNT} borné par la valeur indiquée en couche de base Voir Tableau G.1
Chaussées pour lesquelles la classe de trafic est T2 ou T1 – structures bitumineuses épaisses avec fondation en GNT	
couche de fondation *(GNT subdivisée en sous-couches de 0,25 m d'épaisseur)*	E_{GNT} {1} = 3 $E_{plateforme-support}$ E_{GNT} {sous-couche i} = 3 E_{GNT} {sous-couche (i-1)} E_{GNT} borné par 360 MPa
Chaussées à structure inverse (GNT de type B)	
	E_{GNT} = 480 MPa

IV.2.4.1.2 Materials treated with hydrocarbon binders :

The NF EN 13108 series of standards defines the composition of bituminous mixes on the basis of general characteristics such as grading, voids content, water resistance and resistance to permanent deformation, supplemented by empirical or fundamental characteristics. Two approaches are thus defined: the empirical approach and the fundamental approach.

Additional features are determined by the approach adopted:

- ✓ Empirical" characteristics: These involve specifying a minimum bitumen content for the mix (expressed as a percentage of the total asphalt mass), describing the type of binder, and delimiting the grading ranges using characteristic sieves.

- ✓ Fundamental" characteristics: These are based on measurements of modulus of rigidity and fatigue strength.

Bituminous gravels are classified into three performance classes and two categories according to their grain size (0/14 or 0/20). They can be classified according to the empirical or fundamental approach, as set out in standard NF EN 13108-1.

- ✓ *Empirical approach :*

The modulus values used in the design calculations are given in Table 6.

Table 6 Characteristics to be taken into account when sizing EB-GBs[13]

	Classe	2	3
Valeurs conventionnelles de calcul	Module à 15 °C – 10 Hz ou 0,02 s (MPa)	9 000	9 000
	ε_6 (µdéf)	80	90
	– 1/b	5	5
	S_N	0,3	0,3
	k_c	1,3	1,3

✓ ***Fundamental approach :***

In the fundamental approach, the foreword to asphalt standard NF EN 13108-1 sets minimum values for modulus E and strain ε6 (at 10°C and 25 Hz) by material class, as shown in Table 7. These values are used to make a preliminary estimate before obtaining laboratory test results on the material in question.

Characteristics in excess of these minimum values for modulus E and fatigue characteristic ε6 may be taken into account in the design, provided that these characteristics have been obtained during the formulation study on materials made with site components, with the prescribed percentage of voids. However, these characteristics must not exceed the maximum values defined for the class in question.

Table 7 Minimum and maximum mechanical properties of EB-GB to be retained for dimensioning within the framework of the fundamental approach[13]

	Classe	2	3	4
Valeurs minimales	Module à 15 °C – 10 Hz ou 0,02 s (MPa)	9 000	9 000	11 000
	ε_6 (µdéf)	80	90	100
Valeurs maximales	Module à 15 °C – 10 Hz ou 0,02 s (MPa)	11 000	11 000	14 000
	ε_6 (µdéf)	90	100	115
Valeurs à appliquer forfaitairement	– 1/b	5	5	5
	S_N	0,3	0,3	0,3
	k_c	1,3	1,3	1,3

IV.2.4.2 Comparison of calculated stresses in the structure and permissible stresses :

The estimated load for each layer at risk of deterioration, whether due to flexural fatigue or permanent deformation, must be less than or equal to the absolute allowable load. If this condition is not met, the calculation is repeated by adjusting the thickness of the layers or modifying the materials used in the pavement structure or subgrade, until all the design criteria are satisfied.

41

IV.2.5 Structural design to withstand the effects of freezing and thawing :

Structural design of road pavements to withstand freeze-thaw in accordance with standard NF P 98-086[13]is carried out by applying the following approach (illustrated in Figure 22) :

- ✓ Selection of the reference winter, characterized by its frost index IR, against which the pavement is to be protected.
- ✓ Determination of the permissible frost quantity at subgrade level QPF, based on the soil in place, the subgrade selected and the mechanical strength of the pavement. The corresponding frost index, It, is equal to the square of QPF.
- ✓ Calculation of the permissible surface frost index IS from It and a heat transfer model through the upper pavement layers.
- ✓ Calculation of the permissible atmospheric frost index IA as a function of IS.
- ✓ Comparison between AI and IR.

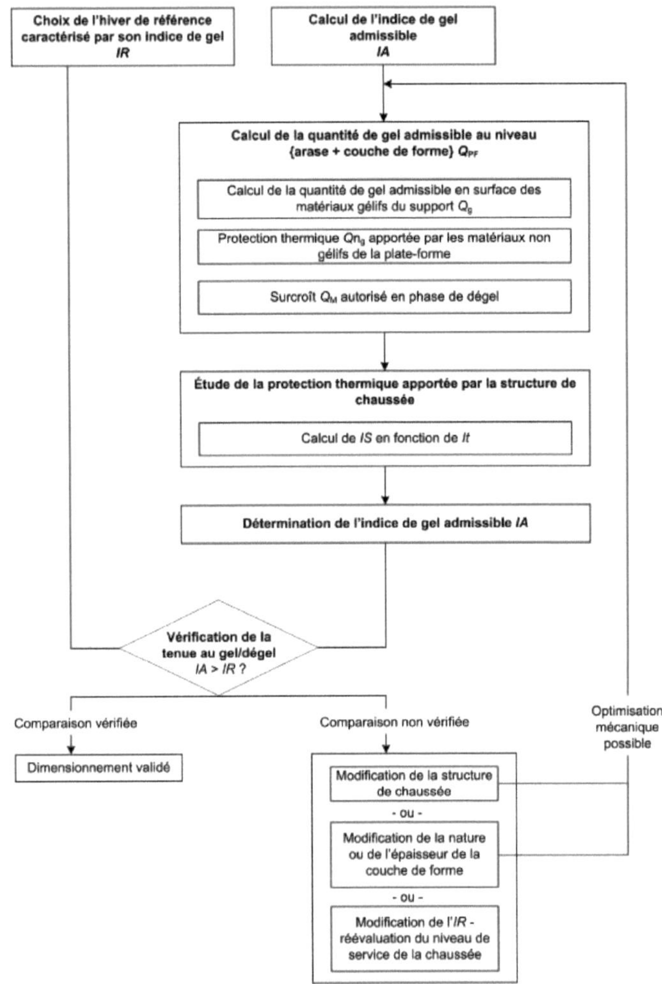

Figure 22Freeze-thaw verification principle[13]

IV.2.5.1 Reference winter :

The reference winter is a specific period chosen to assess the freeze/thaw conditions to which a pavement will be exposed. It is characterized by its frost index (RI), which represents the most unfavorable frost conditions expected during this period. This period can be determined on the basis of historical climate data or weather forecasts for the region where the pavement is located. In general, the reference winter is chosen to represent a season when frost conditions are likely to have a significant impact on the pavement structure.

IV.2.5.2 The permissible atmospheric frost index IA :

The permissible frost index is a measure used in the freeze-thaw verification of pavements to assess their resistance to frost conditions. It represents the amount of frost the pavement can withstand without suffering excessive damage.

To calculate it, several steps are required:

- ❖ **Determining the permissible amount of frost at subgrade level (QPF):** This depends on factors such as the type of soil in place, the subgrade used and the mechanical strength of the pavement. This amount of frost is expressed in terms of deformation or stress, depending on the calculation method chosen.

- ❖ **Calculation of the corresponding frost index (It):** Once the permissible frost quantity has been determined, the frost index (It) is calculated by taking the square of QPF.

- ❖ **Calculating the permissible surface frost index (SFI):** Using a heat transfer model through the upper layers of the pavement, the permissible surface frost index (SFI) is calculated from the frost index (It).

- ❖ **Calculation of the admissible atmospheric frost index (AI):** Based on IS, the admissible atmospheric frost index (AI) is calculated to assess the frost conditions actually encountered on the pavement.

- ❖ **Comparison between IA and IR:** Finally, a comparison is made between the admissible atmospheric frost index (IA) and the reference winter frost index (IR) to assess whether the pavement's freeze/thaw conditions are acceptable.

V.   Formulation of bituminous mixes according to the Moroccan directive for lime mixes:

V.1   The various methods of formulating asphalt mixes :

Over the last four decades, asphalt mix design techniques have progressed to meet the changing needs of customers. This evolution is driven by increasing road traffic, the need to ensure road safety, comfort and durability, and the consideration of various factors such as maintenance and user comfort, in specific climatic conditions and technical context (in particular the design and dimensioning of pavement layers). This evolution has led to a growing complexity in the formulation of materials. Indeed, mix design is becoming increasingly delicate, as any improvement in one characteristic due to a change in composition can have a negative impact on another. For example, increasing binder content can improve fatigue resistance but adversely affect rutting resistance[15].

The properties required of a bituminous material vary according to the layer in which it is used. For base courses, whose main function is to distribute loads on the ground without suffering excessive deformation, the asphalt must be relatively rigid, fatigue-resistant, capable of resisting permanent deformation and fairly compact. On the other hand, for a wearing course that is directly exposed to traffic and climatic conditions, the emphasis is on durability, with good water resistance, as well as resistance to permanent deformation. In addition, surface characteristics such as roughness, rolling noise and photometry are also important. Depending on specific requirements, the wearing course mix must be sufficiently compact to prevent water infiltration into the lower layers, or on the contrary sufficiently permeable to allow water drainage. These multiple requirements can sometimes be contradictory[15].

Approaches to addressing this question are diverse and depend largely on the specific context of each locality, In our analysis, we were able to identify three distinct methods of formulation[15] :

❖   The recipe formulation method :

The recipe method is based on local experience. It consists in reproducing a known composition that has proved its worth under specific conditions of use and over long periods of time. The use of these recipes can sometimes be supplemented by a few tests based on empirical methods.

❖   The empirical testing formulation method :

The most commonly used empirical method is the Marshall method. It involves compressing specimens according to specific protocols, and then comparing the results of the mechanical tests with the behavior observed in the field.

❖   The fundamental test formulation method :

This method incorporates tests whose results can be used directly as input data for dimensioning models. This applies in particular to dynamic modulus and fatigue strength values.

The study of bituminous mix design according to the Moroccan Lime Asphalt Directive can be described as empirical, although it does involve "performance-related" testing, with the aim of assessing the water sensitivity and compaction rate of bituminous pavements. Water resistance tests and Marshall and/or Gyratory Shear Press tests on asphalt mixes are scheduled as part of the mix design study [4].

V.2   Definitions and principles of tests used in asphalt mix design trials :

V.2.1   The Gyratory Shear Press[16]

The hydrocarbon mixture, prepared in the laboratory, is placed in a cylindrical mold with a diameter of 150 mm or 160 mm, at test temperature (approx. 130°C to 160°C). A vertical pressure of 0.6 MPa is applied to the top of the specimen. At the same time, the specimen is slightly tilted at a shallow angle of around 1° (external) or 0.82° (internal) and subjected to a circular motion, resulting in compaction by kneading. The increase in compactness (and decrease in the percentage of voids) is observed as a function of the number of gyrations performed.

The test is used to assess the rate of asphalt compaction on site, for a given number of gyrations, depending on the type of asphalt, the nature of the aggregate and the thickness of the mix.

V.2.2   Water resistance[17]

Water resistance is usually measured by means of the Duriez test within the framework of Moroccan standardization. The principle of the test is to compact the hydrocarbon mix in a cylindrical mold using double-acting static pressure. One part of the test specimens is kept without immersion at controlled temperature (18°C) and hygrometry, while the other part is kept immersed. Each group of specimens is crushed in single compression.

Water resistance is assessed by the ratio of resistance after immersion to resistance when dry.

V.2.3   The rutting test[15]

The test body is a 5 cm or 10 cm thick parallelepiped plate, depending on the thickness of the asphalt mix, which may be less or greater than 5 cm. This plate is exposed to traffic from a wheel fitted with a tire, with a frequency of 1 Hz, a load of 5 kN and a pressure of 6 bar, under rigorous temperature conditions (60°C).

Interpretation: The depth of deformation generated by the passage of the wheel is measured as a function of the number of cycles. Specific criteria relate to a percentage of rutting at a given number of cycles, which depends on the type of material and its class.

V.2.4   Module tests[15]

Mixture stiffness is assessed either by a complex modulus test, involving sinusoidal loading on a trapezoidal or parallelepiped specimen, or by a uniaxial tensile test, performed on a cylindrical or parallelepiped specimen. The load is applied in a range of small deformations, with control of time or frequency, temperature and loading law.

The modulus, expressing the ratio of stress to strain, is calculated for each elementary test. Using time-temperature equivalence, a master modulus curve is plotted at a given temperature. This allows us to understand the behavior of the mixture over a wide range of load times and frequencies.

Specifications refer to the module at 15°C and a frequency of 10 Hz, or a charge time of 0.02 s.

V.2.5   Fatigue strength[15]

A trapezoidal specimen is subjected to an imposed deformation at a fixed temperature and loading frequency. When the stress required to maintain the strain constant is halved, the specimen is considered damaged at the specified number of cycles. On an lg/lg graph, the different couples (loading level, number of cycles to damage) are placed along a fatigue line. At 10^6 cycles, the loading threshold on the straight line represents the characteristic fatigue strength value: ε6.

V.2.6   Definitions and relationships useful for formulation studies :

V.2.6.1   Binder content

In the formulation study, two terms are used to express binder content: external binder content (TLext), which indicates the proportion of binder mass to dry aggregate mass, in accordance withEquation 8or the internal binder content (tlint), which expresses the proportion of the binder mass to the total mass of the mix.[15]as defined in The relationship between the two is expressed byEquation 10 :

Equation 8external binder content

$$TL_{ext} = 100 \times \frac{Masse\ de\ bitume}{Masse\ de\ granulats\ secs}$$

Equation 9Internal binder content

$$tl_{int} = 100 \times \frac{Masse\ de\ bitume}{Masse\ de\ granulats\ secs + Masse\ de\ bitume}$$

Equation 10relationship between external and internal binder content

$$TL_{ext} = \frac{100 \times tl_{int}}{100 - tl_{int}}$$

V.2.6.2   Richness module K

The richness modulus, K, is a quantity that is proportional to the conventional thickness of the hydrocarbon binder film covering the aggregate.[15]. This K value is related to the external binder content by the following equationEquation 11 as follows

Equation 11Wealth modulus K

$$TL_{ext} = K \times \alpha \sqrt[5]{\Sigma}$$

where Σ is the specific surface area, expressed in square metres per kilogram, determined by the relationship :

$$\Sigma = 0.20g + 2.2S + 12s + 135f, \text{ in m}^2/\text{kg},$$

With :

- ✓ g, proportions of elements greater than 6mm
- ✓ S, element proportions between 6 and 0.315mm
- ✓ s, element proportions between 0.315 and 0.08mm
- ✓ f, proportions of elements smaller than 0.08mm
- ✓ a: correction coefficient proportions, designed to take into account the density of the aggregates. If this density is equal to 2.65g/cm3, a=1. Otherwise, a=2.65/aggregate density.

V.2.6.3 Percentage of voids or Compactness :

❖ **Real density :**

The actual density can be calculated from the component densities and is denoted MVRc [15] and calculated from the following equations:

Equation 12Calculated actual density

$$MVRc = \frac{Masse\ de\ granulats + Masse\ de\ bitume}{Vg + Vb}$$

External bitumen content :

Equation 13:Real density with TLext

$$MVRc = \frac{100 \cdot TL_{ext}}{\dfrac{\%G_1}{\rho_{g1}} + \dfrac{\%G_2}{\rho_{g2}} + \ldots + \dfrac{\%G_n}{\rho_{gn}} + \dfrac{TL_{ext}}{\rho_b}}$$

❖ **Apparent density :**

Apparent density is obtained by dividing the mass of the sample by its apparent volume. The latter can be determined by geometric measurement (MVA) or hydrostatic weighing, with or without kerosene (NF EN 12697-6).

❖ **Percentage of voids and compactness :**

Compactness and percentage of voids are determined from measurements of real density *MVR* and apparent density *MVA* and by the following relationships[15] :

$$C\% = 100 \times MVA/ MVR$$
$$v\% = 100\ (1 - (MVA/ MVR))$$

The compactness *C%* and the percentage of voids *v%* are related by the following equation:

$$100\% = C\% + v\%.$$

V.2.7 Mix design test :

Based on components such as aggregates, fines, hydrocarbon binders and mineral additives, which are identified and representative of the materials to be used in the project, a series of laboratory tests is carried out to characterize the behavior of a hydrocarbon mix. The choice of test sequence depends on the test level required by the client, ranging from 1 to 4. This level is generally determined by factors such as the type of mix, the position of the layer in the pavement, its thickness, the expected traffic, the specific stresses, the purpose of the layer, the nature of the lower layers and the size of the worksite. The mix design test also includes specifications concerning constituents, mix composition, sample preparation and main material performances.

V.2.7.1   Sand specifications :

As a general rule, in Morocco, the sand fraction used in the manufacture of hot mix asphalt is 0/4, with a minimum fines content of 12%. According to the recommendations of the[5] sand **cleanliness** is assessed using the sand equivalent test, where results must exceed the limit value, set at 30% for bitumen gravel and 40% for bituminous mixes.

Other tests are recommended by asphalt mix manufacturing standards. Among these, the **angularity** test (NF EN 933-6) is specified when the mix is intended for wearing courses. Results must generally fall within the ECS35 or 38 categories, except for asphalt mixes based on semi-compacted bituminous concrete (EB-BBS), for which the ECS30 category is accepted.

V.2.7.2   Gravel specifications :

❖ Granularity :

For chippings, the granular fractions usually used are: 2/4, 2/6, 4/6, 4/10, 6/10, 10/14.

For asphalt mixes intended for base courses, fractions 2/10, 6/14, 6/20, 10/20 and 14/20 can also be used.

❖ Form :

According to the recommendations of the directive[5] shape is assessed using the flattening coefficient test, where results must be below the limit value, set at 20% for gravel with a fraction greater than or equal to 10 mm and 25% for gravel with a fraction between 4mm-10mm.

❖ Hardness

According to the recommendations of the directive[5] hardness is assessed using the Los Angles and Micro-Deval tests:

- ✓ LA < 30 for bitumen gravel
- ✓ LA < 25 for asphalt mixes.
- ✓ M.D.E < 25 for bitumen gravel
- ✓ M.D.E < 20 for asphalt mixes.

Compensation between Los Angeles and MDE values may be allowed up to a maximum of 5 points.

❖ Angularity

Angularity is only checked when the source material is alluvial. In the case of solid rock mining, the material is naturally crushed and considered pure crushed.

Table 8Angularity specifications[5]

Nature de Matériau	Trafic	Angularité
G.B.B	T0	R.C≥4 concassé pur
0/20	T1	IC≥100% (RC=1)
et	T2	IC≥50%
0/25	T3 et T4	IC≥20%
B.B 0/10 et 0/14	toutes catégories	R.C≥4 concassé pur

V.2.7.3   Binder specifications :

As a general rule, in Morocco, grade 35/50 bitumen is most often used, with the following specifications:

test title	methods	*Specifications*
Needle penetrability of pure bitumens in (10ieme of mm)	NM EN 1426[3]	35-50
Determination of softening point in (°C)	NM EN 1427[4]	50-58
Determination : - flash point. - of the fire point in an open vessel	NM ISO 2592[18]	>240 -

V.2.7.4   Mixture composition specifications :

The composition of the asphalt mix must comply with the road CPC specifications and the hot mix manufacturing guidelines, which are summarized as follows:

❖ **Aggregate mix properties and binder type :**

The table below shows the pass intervals for different sieves, establishing a range within which the average value should lie. On the other hand, for each method (EB or GBB), it recalls the classes of pure bitumen to be used.

Table 9Aggregate mix properties and binder type[5]

Granularité % Passant au Tamis de (mm)	EB 0/10 Roulement	EB 0/14 Liaison	GBB	
			0/20	0/25
25	-	-	-	100
20	-	-	100	74-100
14	-	100	-	-
10	100	-	-	-
6	65-80	50-65	44-65	37-60
2	30-45	25-38	25-42	24-40
0,08	5 - 9	4 - 8	6-10	6-10
Bitume	40/50 ou 60/70 ou 80/100	40/50 ou 60/70		

❖ **Characterization tests :**

A set of specifications has been developed to assess compaction behavior and mechanical properties, in particular water resistance, as illustrated in the table below. These performances are assessed by means of tests that constitute the minimum study, according to the CPC routier and the Moroccan directive for lime mixes, to be carried out in order to approve a mix design and select the various parameters.

In addition, to assess the compaction capacity of an asphalt mix design using the PCG test, the following conditions are considered according to the Moroccan directive for lime mixes: a compactness of less than 89% after 10 rotations, a compactness of 92 to 96% after 60 rotations for the EB 0/10 mix, and a compactness of 96% after 80 rotations for the EB 0/14 mix.

Table 10Test specifications for asphalt mix design tests[5]

		EB 0/10 ROULEMENT	EB 0/14 LIAISON	GBB 0/20 et 0/25
Module de richesse :				
K		3,45 à 3,9	3,45 à 3,9	2 à 2,5
Essai Marshall :				
- compacité %		93 - 97	92 - 96	91 - 97
- stabilité	40/50	> 1000	> 900	> 800
(bitume)	60/700	> 1000	> 900	> 700
(Kg)	80/100	> 950	> 850	-
Fluage (mm)		< 4	< 4	
Essai L.P.C :		90 à 95	88 à 94	88 à 95
- compacité %				
- compression bras				
	40/50	> 60	> 60	> 50
(bitume) 80/100	60/700	> 55	> 55	> 45
	80/100	> 50	> 45	-
RH/RS		> 0,75		> 0,65

V.2.7.5   Lime mix design study

Depending on the intended use, the type of asphalt and the stresses to which it will be subjected, requirements may vary. This is why the formulation test has been subdivided into several levels, ranging from 1 to 4, as illustrated in the following figure :

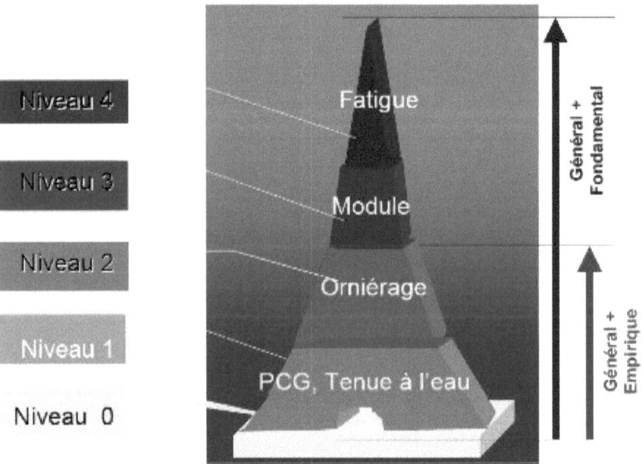

Figure 23Formulation study level[15]

- ❖ **Level 1**: The mix must comply with a range of void percentages in the Gyratory Shear Press test, as well as the defined water resistance criterion.
- ❖ **Level 2**: This level includes the tests from level 1 (Gyratory Shear Press and water resistance), plus a rutting test.
- ❖ **Level 3**: This level includes the Gyratory Shear Press and water resistance tests of level 1, the rutting test of level 2, and the characterization of the mix modulus. The modulus test is prescribed for large-scale projects and when the layer in question contributes to the structural performance of the pavement.
- ❖ **Level 4**: This level includes the Gyratory Shear Press and water resistance tests of level 1, the rutting test of level 2, and the modulus characterization of the mix of level 3. It is also enhanced by fatigue strength determination. Fatigue testing is required for very large projects and whenever the layer concerned is subject to fatigue stresses.

V.2.7.6   Estimated duration of a formulation test :

Estimated duration of a formulation test and quantity of materials required, according to the LPC Formulation Manual [15] are shown in the following table:

*Table 11 Estimated duration of a formulation test **and** quantity of materials required[15]*

Niveau d'épreuve	Essai	Quantité de matériau	Durée		Durée globale incluant la préparation
			Essai	Préparation et opérations connexes	
Préparation	Masse volumique réelle du mélange	5 kg pour le mélange	1 j	séchage + essai	2 j
Identification des constituants	Analyse granulométrique	3 kg par fraction granulaire	1 j	séchage + essai	2 j
1	ITSR Méthode B en compression	20 kg (Φ 80) 40 kg (Φ 120)	8 j	séchage + mélange + essai	10 j
	Presse à Cisaillement Giratoire	30 kg	1 j	séchage + mélange + essai	2 j
Total niveau 1		40 kg à 60 kg			12 j
2	Orniérage (2 plaques) Grand-Modèle	50 kg	2 pl. 30 000 cycles 3j	confection + mûrissement + MVa + essai	7 j
Total niveau 2		110 kg			15 j
3	Module en traction directe	80 kg	3 températures 3 ou 4 temps de charge 4 j	confection+ carottage mûrissement + MVa + collage + essai	21 j
	Module complexe	80 kg	1 températures 3 ou 4 fréquences 4 j	confection + sciage mûrissement + MVa + collage + essai	18 j
Total niveau 3		200 kg			21 j
4	Fatigue Trapézoïdale 2 points	200 kg	15 j	confection + sciage + mûrissement + Mva + collage + essai	25 j
Total niveau 4		400 kg			30 j

We would like to stress that these times are estimates, as they do not take into account possible failures in the results of certain tests, as well as material identification tests carried out before the start of asphalt characterization tests, and the laboratory's workload schedule.

Formulation study according to the Moroccan directive for hot mix asphalt materials [5] is carried out according to the procedure illustrated in the figure below:

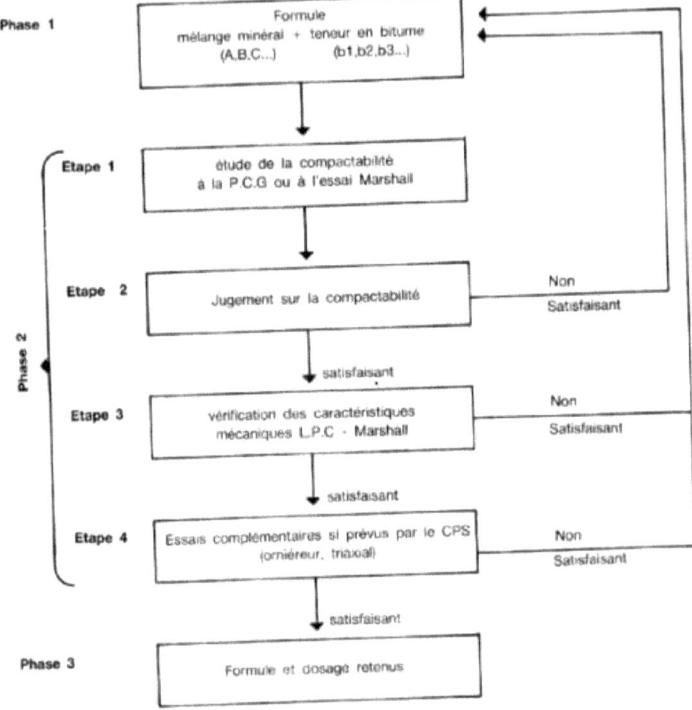

Figure 24Flow chart of the formulation test specimen [5]

VI. Assessment of road pavement condition using indirect prospecting methods :

Despite the efforts made during the preliminary dimensioning and design phases to mitigate the effects of climatic and mechanical stresses, as well as the precautionary measures incorporated into the road design project, infrastructures such as nozzles, drains, concrete ditches and other hydraulic structures are planned to allow drainage of surface water and weathering. These measures are designed to reduce climatic stresses, ensuring efficient water drainage and minimizing the risks associated with water-sensitive asphalt pavements. In this way, they help to increase the durability and resistance of road pavements in a wide range of weather conditions.

However, despite these precautions, road pavements are subject to deterioration, hence the importance of assessing their condition using indirect prospecting methods. These methods are essential for anticipating preventive maintenance needs. In this section, we look at some of the methods used in the road sector to assess pavement condition and anticipate maintenance requirements.

VI.1 Pavement deflection under load :

Pavement deflection under load refers (13t axle) to the bending or deformation a pavement undergoes in response to an applied load, such as the passage of a vehicle or heavy equipment. This deflection is measured using deflection tests such as the Falling Weight Deflectometer (FWD) or the Benkelman Beam, as illustrated in the photos below.

When a load is applied to the pavement, it deflects or deforms under the effect of the pressure exerted. Deflection is measured by recording the vertical distance between a fixed reference point on the pavement and the pavement surface under load. This measurement is used to assess the stiffness of the pavement, as well as its ability to support the load and resist permanent deformation.

Deflection is not very sensitive to variations in the modulus of the pavement materials, but it is sensitive to variations in thickness and very sensitive to variations in the bearing capacity of the subgrade.

Pavement deflection under load is an important indicator of pavement performance. It is used to assess pavement bearing capacity, detect areas of weakness or deterioration, and guide maintenance and repair decisions to ensure road safety and durability.

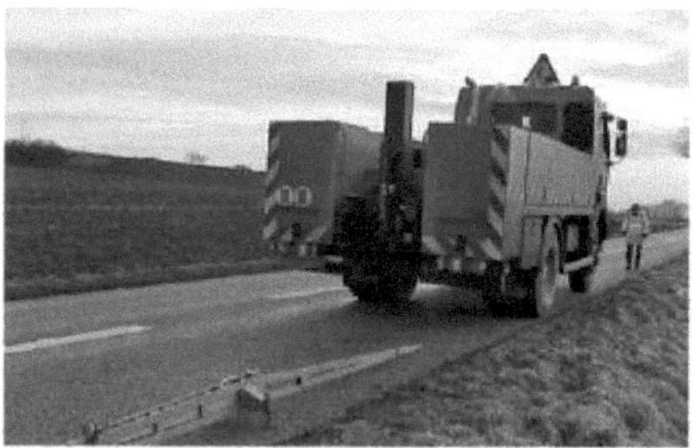

Figure 25 Benkelman beam[19]

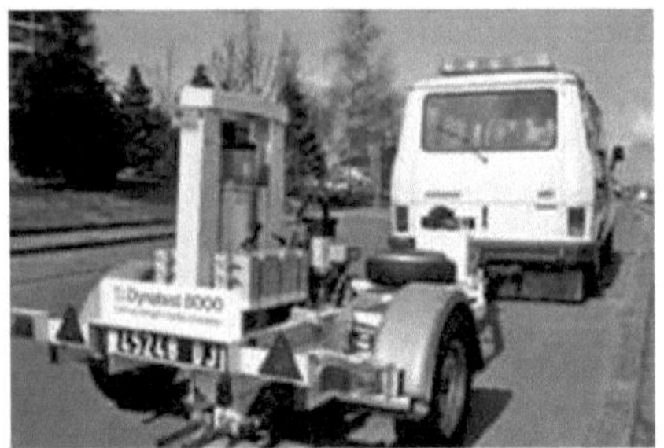

Figure 26:Photo 10 - FWD (Falling Weight Deflectometer)[19]

VI.1.1   Deflection class :

The characteristic deflection value is an indicator of the mechanical behavior of the pavement structure and support. This parameter, which depends on the type of pavement, is generally associated with a deflection class.

Deflections measured with a Lacroix deflectograph under a 13T axle give the following results:

- ✓ Dm in 1/100 mm average section deflection.
- ✓ σ standard deviation around Dm.

The characteristic deflection is then determined using the following equation:

- ✓ D90: Dm + 1.3 s
- ✓ Homogeneity coefficient = σ /Dm

The sections are then classified according to the table below, using the higher of the two measurements (on the axis or on the bank).

Table 12Deflection class[20]

D_{90} en 1/100 mm sur la trace la plus élevée	< 100	100 à 150	150 à 200	> 200
Classe Di	D_1	D_2	D_3	D_4

- ✓ If σ /Dm>0.35, we move up one class.

VI.1.2   Example of the results of a deflection measurement campaign :

The results presented in the table provided by the Road Directorate below represent deflection measurements on the RN 4 national road between kilometre point 100+000 and kilometre point 102+872.

Table 13RN 4 deflection November 2023

Route	ZONE	Abscisse-D (m)	Abscisse-F (m)	PKD	PKF	AXE			RIVE			MAX Axe-Rive	Coefficient d'homogénéité (σ/m)	Classe de déflexion
						MOYENNE	ECART-TYPE (σ)	D90=m+1.3σ	MOYENNE	ECART-TYPE (σ)	D90=m+1.3σ			
N4	Zone 1	0,0	338,3	100,000	100,338	26,1	11,7	41,3	32,8	24,2	64,3	64,3	0,738	D2
N4	Zone 2	338,3	406,1	100,338	100,406	35,6	13,0	52,5	130,4	26,0	164,2	164,2	0,199	D3
N4	Zone 3	406,1	543,5	100,406	100,544	32,4	14,4	51,2	48,3	15,0	67,8	67,8	0,311	D1
N4	Zone 4	543,5	1313,9	100,544	101,377	19,2	12,2	35,0	27,9	14,8	47,1	47,1	0,530	D2
N4	Zone 5	1313,9	1696,6	101,377	101,760	29,2	15,0	48,7	45,4	17,5	68,2	68,2	0,385	D2
N4	Zone 6	1696,6	1934,8	101,760	101,998	21,7	18,0	45,0	20,0	11,6	35,1	45,0	0,829	D2
N4	Zone 7	1934,8	2483,8	101,998	102,547	26,5	17,6	49,4	42,5	19,2	67,4	67,4	0,452	D2
N4	Zone 8	2483,8	2809,0	102,547	102,872	21,8	11,8	37,1	8,8	13,9	26,9	37,1	0,541	D2

NB :

- ✓ **Abs** : Abscisse.
- ✓ **m.** : moyenne.
- ✓ **(σ)** : ECART-TYPE.
- ✓ **(σ/m)** Coefficient d'homogénéité.

VI.1.3 Georadar (GPR)

Georadar pavement condition assessment (GPR) is an advanced, non-destructive method widely used in the road industry. It is based on the use of high-frequency electromagnetic waves that are emitted through the pavement surface and propagate through the various soil layers. When these waves encounter an interface between two materials of differing electrical conductivity, such as the different layers of pavement, some of the energy is reflected upwards towards the georadar antenna. By measuring the travel time of these reflected waves, as well as their amplitude, the georadar can produce a cross-sectional image of the pavement, showing variations in the composition, thickness and condition of the different layers.

This method offers several significant advantages. Firstly, it enables a rapid and efficient assessment of pavement condition, without the need for excavation work or interruption of road traffic. In addition, it provides detailed data on the internal structure of the pavement, enabling early detection of defects such as cracks, voids, areas of water saturation and material degradation, before they become major problems requiring costly repairs. In addition, georadar can be used to measure the thickness of different pavement layers, which is essential for assessing the pavement's load-bearing capacity and planning any necessary renovation or reinforcement work.

What's more, the use of georadar enables data to be collected over long sections of pavement in a short space of time, making it an extremely effective tool for large-scale road monitoring and maintenance programs. The data collected can be analyzed and interpreted by road engineers to establish preventive maintenance plans and optimize the allocation of budgetary resources, thus helping to extend pavement life and ensure the safety of road users. In short, georadar-based road pavement condition assessment is a valuable and versatile method that plays an essential role in the efficient management of road infrastructures.

VI.1.3.1 Frequencies used :

An increase in frequency leads to more accurate detection but at a limited depth, while a decrease in frequency enables greater depths to be explored at the expense of signal quality.

Table 14 GPR usage characteristics as a function of frequency[21].

Low frequency	High frequency
Large depth	Low depth
Low resolution	High resolution
Geology & geophysics	Pavements and bridge decks

For road applications, the appropriate frequency is between 1 GHz and 2 GHz for a penetration of 0.5m to 1m.

VI.1.3.2 Estimated pavement layer thicknesses :

The GPR system calculates the time required for the wave to travel through each material interface. To evaluate the thickness of the layers, it is necessary to know the propagation velocity in each material, determined by the formula :

$$V = \frac{c}{\sqrt{\varepsilon_r}}$$

With :

- ✓ c: speed of light.
- ✓ ε_r relative dielectric permittivity of the material.

For road materials, we have orders of magnitude of Ɛr, but these vary considerably depending on the presence of water.

Table 15 Orders of magnitude of the relative dielectric permittivity of the material [21].

Material	Ɛr
Dry asphalt	2 - 5
Wet asphalt	6 - 12
Dry concrete	4 - 8
Wet concrete	8 - 15
Bitumen	2,7
Dry sand	2,5 - 6
Wet sand	10 - 25
Ice	2,5 - 4
Dry soil	4 - 10
Wet soil	10 - 30
Frozen ground	4 - 8
Dry limestone	7
Wet limestone	8

VI.2 Electric tomography :

Evaluating the condition of road pavements using electrical tomography is an advanced method that provides detailed information on the condition of the soil supporting the pavement. Electrical tomography is based on the principle of measuring the electrical resistivity of materials using electrodes placed along the pavement surface.

This method involves injecting electric current into the ground through a series of electrodes placed along the pavement. Variations in electrical resistance in the soil are measured using receiver electrodes placed at specific positions. These measurements are then used to reconstruct a cross-sectional image of the pavement, showing variations in electrical conductivity at different depths.

The main advantage of electrical tomography is its ability to provide detailed information on the distribution of materials and structures beneath the pavement surface, including areas of water saturation, voids, areas of compaction and layers of materials with different electrical conductivities. This enables early detection of defects and potential damage, such as cracks, subsidence and material degradation, before they become major problems requiring costly repairs.

What's more, electrical tomography can be carried out on long sections of pavement in a short space of time, making it an effective tool for large-scale road monitoring and maintenance programs. The data collected can be analyzed and interpreted by road engineers to establish preventive maintenance plans and optimize the allocation of budgetary resources.

In short, assessing the condition of road pavements using electrical tomography is a valuable method for detecting defects and potential damage at an early stage, helping to extend pavement life and ensure the safety of road users.

VI.2.1 Theoretical foundations and principles :

Artificially generated electrical currents are injected into the ground, and the resulting potential variations are measured. The profiles of these variations provide information on the nature and electrical characteristics of the various underground structures. The greater the electrical difference between the main soil structure and the heterogeneities, the easier it is to detect them. Thus, soil electrical resistivity can be used as an indicator of the diversity of soil physical properties [22].

❖ The resistivity ρ (Ω.m) and defined according to the following equation:

Equation 14Resistivity calculation

$$\rho = R\left(\frac{S}{L}\right)$$

With :

- ✓ R the electrical resistance (V),
- ✓ L the length of the cylinder (m),
- ✓ S its cross-sectional area (m2).

In a homogeneous, isotropic half-space, the electrical equipotential lines take on a hemispherical shape when the current electrodes are placed on the ground surface, as shown in the figure below. In this case, the current density J (A/m²) must be calculated for all radial directions according to :

Equation 15Current density calculation

$$J = \frac{I}{2\pi r^2}$$

Where $2.\pi.r^2$ is the surface area of a hemispherical sphere of radius r.

❖ The potential V can then be expressed as follows:

Equation 16Current potential calculation

$$V = \frac{\rho I}{2\pi r}$$

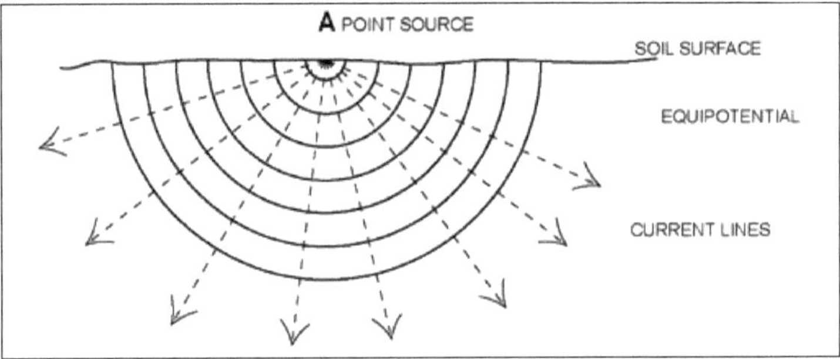

Figure 27Current flow distribution in a homogeneous soil.[22]

❖ To measure electrical resistivity, four electrodes are generally used: two electrodes, A and B, to inject the current (called "current electrodes"), and two other electrodes, M and N, to record the resulting potential difference (called "potential electrodes"). The potential difference ΔV measured between electrodes M and N is given by the following equation:

Equation 17Calculation of current potential difference

$$\Delta V = \frac{\rho I}{2\pi}\left[\frac{1}{AM} - \frac{1}{BM} - \frac{1}{AN} + \frac{1}{BN}\right]$$

Where AM, BM, AN and BN represent the geometric distance between electrodes A and M, B and M, A and N, and B and N, respectively.

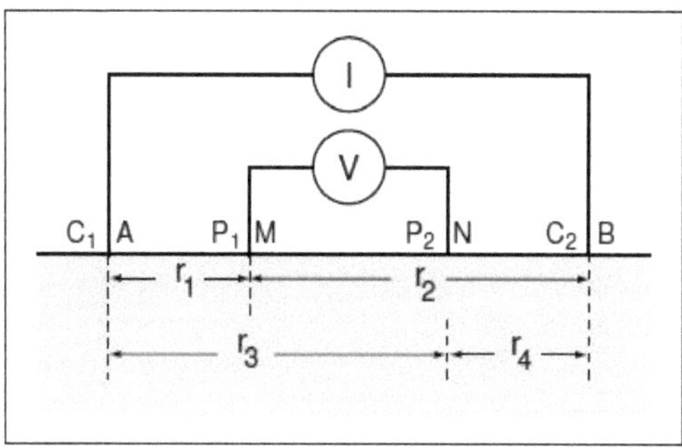

Figure 28Four-electrode surface device.

❖ Electrical resistivity is then calculated using the following formula:

Equation 18Calculation of electrical resistivity

$$\rho = \left[\frac{2\pi}{(1/AM) - (1/BM) - (1/AN) + (1/BN)}\right]\frac{\Delta V}{I}$$

$$= K\frac{\Delta V}{I}$$

Where K is a geometric coefficient that depends on the arrangement of the four electrodes A, B, M and N.

VI.2.2 Variation in electrical resistivity as a function of soil properties :

Electrical resistivity is a function of a number of soil properties, including the nature of the solid constituents (particle size distribution, mineralogy), the arrangement of voids (porosity, pore size distribution, connectivity), the degree of water saturation (water content), the electrical resistivity of the fluid (solute concentration) and temperature. The table below summarizes the typical electrical resistivity ranges of earth materials.

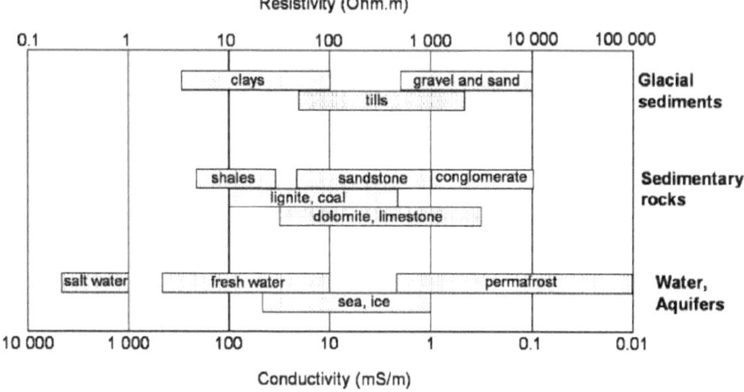

Figure 29 Typical ranges of electrical resistivities of terrestrial materials [22]

VI.2.3 2D electrical tomography :

Two-dimensional multi-electrode arrays provide a vertical representation of the probed medium. Electrodes are moved along a line at regular intervals, recording a resistivity measurement at each step, as illustrated in Figure 30. The data obtained are used to construct resistivity profiles. By progressively increasing the distance between electrodes, a greater depth of investigation is obtained. The data are presented in 2D pseudo-sections, enabling simultaneous visualization of horizontal and vertical variations in resistivity. Different network configurations are used (Figure 31), with different impacts on resolution, sensitivity and depth of investigation. Selection of the configuration depends on the characteristics of the medium to be studied, as illustrated in Figure 32.

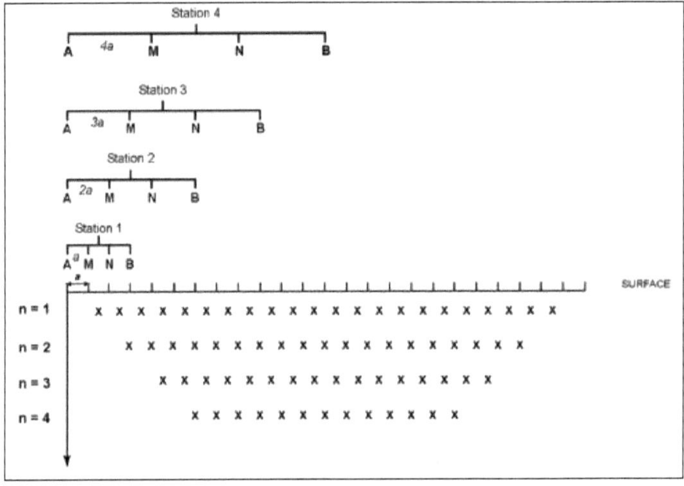

Figure 302D electrical resistivity pseudo-section.[22]

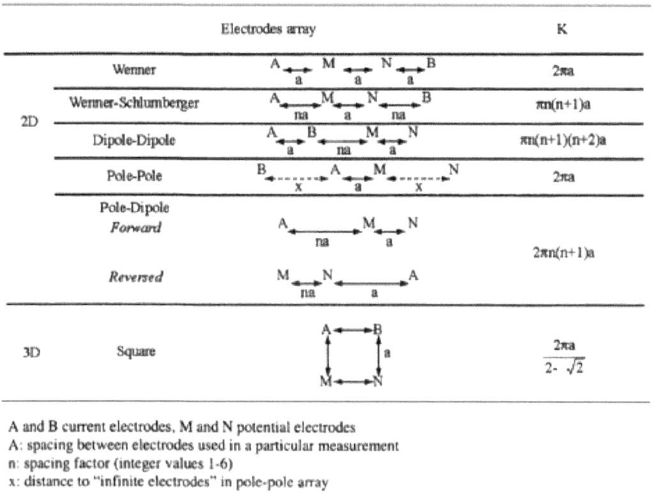

	Electrodes array		K
2D	Wenner	A — M — N — B (a, a, a)	$2\pi a$
	Wenner-Schlumberger	A — M — N — B (na, a, na)	$\pi n(n+1)a$
	Dipole-Dipole	A — B — M — N (a, na, a)	$\pi n(n+1)(n+2)a$
	Pole-Pole	B ---- A — M ---- N (x, a, x)	$2\pi a$
	Pole-Dipole *Forward*	A ——— M — N (na, a)	$2\pi n(n+1)a$
	Reversed	M — N ——— A (na, a)	
3D	Square	A — B / M — N (a)	$\dfrac{2\pi a}{2-\sqrt{2}}$

A and B current electrodes, M and N potential electrodes
A: spacing between electrodes used in a particular measurement
n: spacing factor (integer values 1-6)
x: distance to "infinite electrodes" in pole-pole array

Figure 31Example of a 2D in-line electrode array and 3D electrode device configuration.[22]

	Wenner	Wenner–Schlumberger	Dipole–dipole	Pole–pole	Pole–dipole
Sensitivity of the array horizontal structures	++++	++	+	++	++
Sensitivity of the array vertical structures	+	++	++++	++	+
Depth of investigation	+	++	+++	++++	+++
Horizontal data coverage	+	++	+++	++++	+++
Signal Strength	++++	+++	+	++++	++

The labels are classified form (+) to (++++), equivalent at poor sensitivity to high sensitivity for the different array configurations.

Figure 32Characteristics of different types of 2D network configurations.[22]

VI.2.4 3-D electric tomography ·

Two methods can be used to acquire three-dimensional electrical resistivity:

The first method involves the construction of a 3D electrical image by reconstructing a two-dimensional network of parallel pseudo-sections, thus enabling an accurate image to be recorded when the electrical anomalies are preferentially oriented and the measuring electrodes are perpendicular to these anomalies. Electrode configurations oriented in at least two mutually perpendicular directions are recommended for sites with heterogeneous subsurface conditions.

The second method uses a square array of four electrodes, offering a less orientation-dependent resistivity measurement than in-line arrays.

VI.2.5 The inversion model

All inversion methods are fundamentally focused on creating a model of the subsurface that best reflects the measurements made. This model, mathematically defined, represents the expected response according to the geological conditions encountered. To make this transition from the space of measurements, where we have apparent resistivity values, to the space of the physical parameters of the model to be estimated, such as the resistivity at each point of the section, we call on mathematical tools such as the finite element or finite difference method.

A commonly used software package for this task is res2dinv. This inversion program takes data collected in the field, usually in pseudo-section form, and generates corresponding subsurface resistivity models.

In short, electrical inversion is a complex but essential process that enables us to transform field data into valuable information about the composition and structure of the subsurface.

VII. Damage to wearing courses and crack propagation in asphalt mixes:

The catalog of pavement surface degradations[23]describes a crack as a visible fracture line appearing on the pavement surface. The appearance of cracks on the pavement surface can be attributed to a variety of causes:

- When cracking results from the formation of cracks in the lower layers of the pavement, such as the sub-base layers or the base of the wearing course, which rise up to the pavement surface, this phenomenon is referred to as structural deterioration. In this case, defects in the underlying layers directly affect the pavement surface, compromising its stability and durability.

- On the other hand, when the crack starts at the surface of the pavement and only penetrates the top layer without affecting the underlying layers, we speak of superficial deterioration. This type of cracking can result from a variety of factors, such as thermal stresses, fatigue or freeze-thaw cycles. Although shallower, this type of cracking can nevertheless compromise pavement integrity by allowing water and atmospheric agents to penetrate the underlying layers, thus accelerating the deterioration process.

In short, the distinction between structural and superficial crack degradation in pavements is important for understanding degradation mechanisms and developing appropriate maintenance and repair strategies. Effective crack management is essential to ensure the durability and safety of roads and freeways.

VII.1 Different types of pavement damage :

VII.1.1 Deformations:

❖ **Bank** subsidence :

Settling of the pavement at the edge, sometimes forming a depression accompanied by a bead of material along the pavement, as illustrated in the figure below. Possible causes of this deformation include pavement fatigue due to insufficient material thickness or quality, as well as insufficient edge shoring. This deterioration is often exacerbated by the presence of water trapped in the depression.

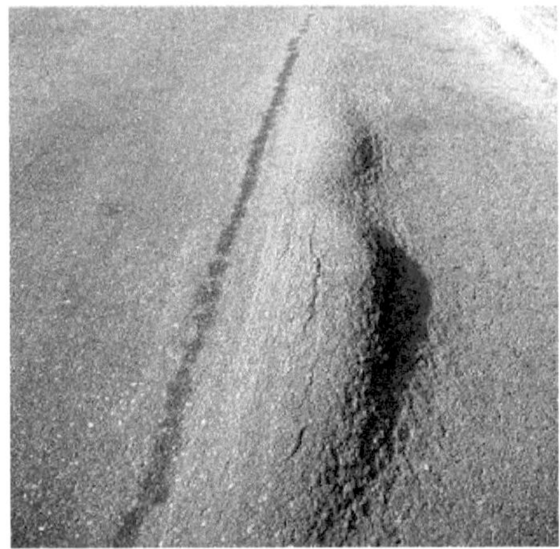

Figure 33Bank subsidence accompanied by bead formation[24]

❖ Flache:

Settlement in the middle of the pavement, often in a rounded shape, as illustrated in the figure below. The possible cause of this deformation in the case of flexible pavements is fatigue due to a localized bearing capacity defect in the soil, such as a pocket of wet clay.

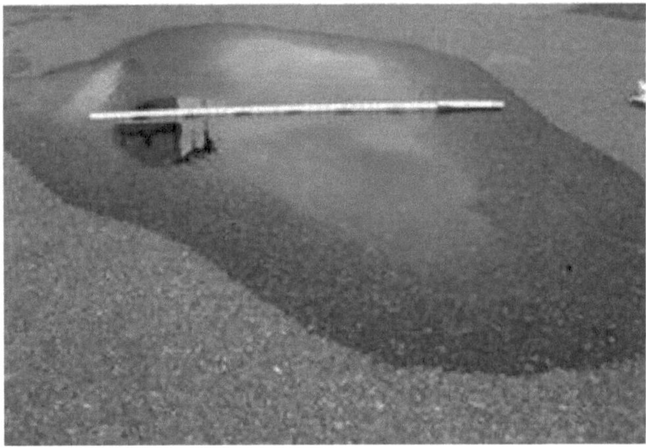

Figure 34Depression in asphalt pavement[24]

❖ Rutting :

The possible causes of this deformation are either pavement fatigue due to compaction of the lower layers caused by a lack of bearing capacity of the soil (large-radius rutting), or poor stability of a flexible pavement on steep slopes, ramps or braking zones (small-radius rutting).

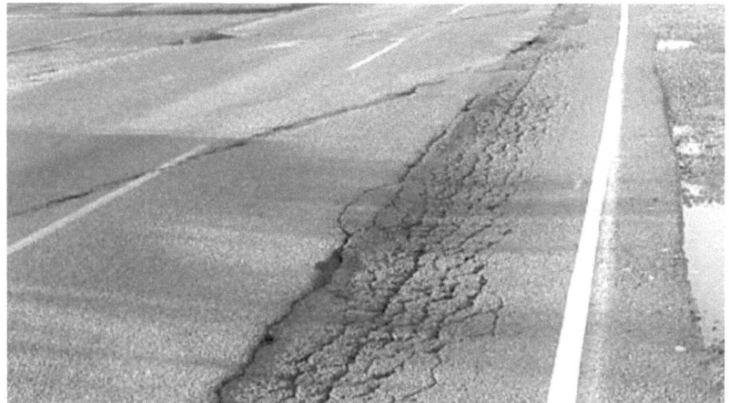

Figure 35Rutting of asphalt pavement. [24]

VII.1.2 Cracks:

❖ Longitudinal crack :

Longitudinal cracks form in the direction of traffic or mainly parallel to the pavement axis, as shown in the figure below. Possible causes of these cracks are poorly constructed paving joints, shrinkage of the asphalt layer, daily temperature cycles, cracks in an underlying layer that are reflected in the pavement, and longitudinal segregation, caused by incorrect paver operation.

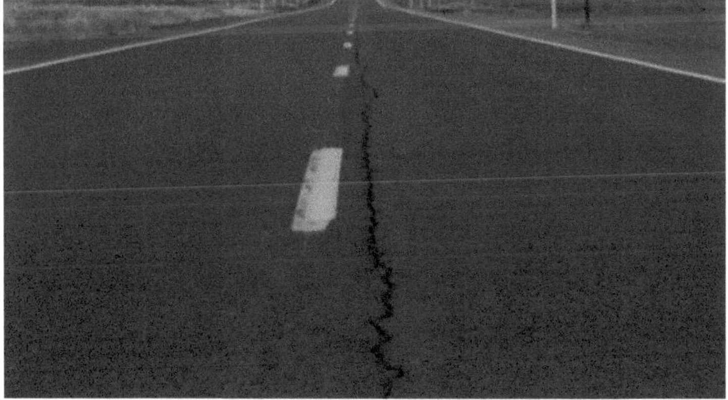

Figure 36 Longitudinal crack in the pavement[24]

❖ Transverse cracks :

Transverse cracks are mainly perpendicular to the pavement axis or paving direction, as shown in the figure below. Possible causes of transverse cracking are surface shrinkage of the hot mix material due to low temperatures, or hardening of the bituminous binder.

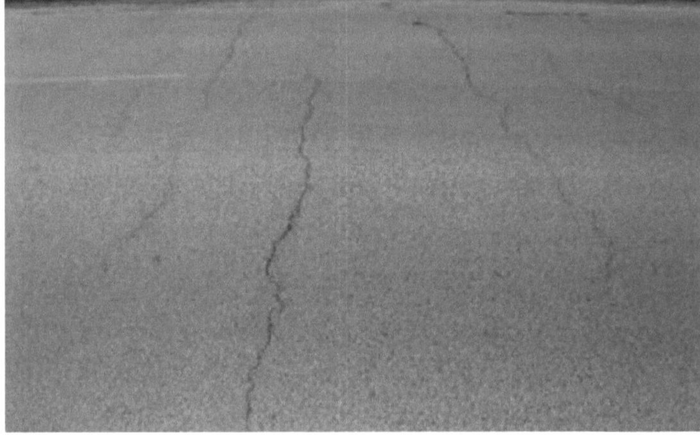

Figure 37Transverse crack in pavement[24]

❖ Crazing :

A series of more or less closely spaced cracks forming a mesh, as shown in the figure below. Possible causes Extreme weather conditions and heavily loaded vehicles are the main causes of fatigue cracks and/or a weak, thin wearing course and base layer also contribute to the appearance of cracks. These cracks can lead to structural failure and water infiltration through the cracks, which can then degrade to form potholes.

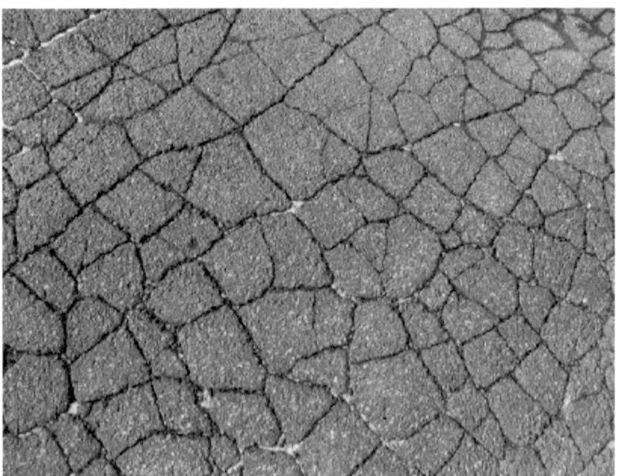

Figure 38:Cracking of asphalt pavement[24]

VII.1.3 Pullouts:

❖ Pothole:

Potholes are bowl-shaped depressions in the road surface, as shown in the figure below. They generally vary in size and have irregular edges. They develop on roads with a thin wearing course. They are generally caused by increased cracking. They are a major cause of accidents, particularly in poor visibility conditions. Potholes also cause further deterioration by collecting rainwater, which seeps directly into the sub-base layer. Possible causes of potholes are as follows:

- ✓ Ongoing deterioration such as thawing of a frozen platform or cracking.
- ✓ Weak points in the base or sub-base layer.

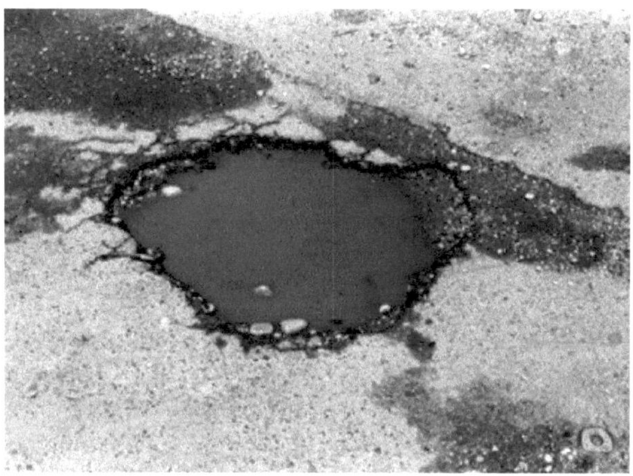

Figure 39 Pothole in asphalt pavement[24]

❖ Pelade:

Peeling is the tearing away of the surface layer in whole patches, as shown in the figure below. Possible causes include defects in the bond coat, such as no bond coat, underdosing, inappropriate choice of binder type, incorrect binder dosage and improper binder preparation. Weather conditions during application can also play a role. In addition, an excessively deformable substrate or excessive stresses at the interface can contribute to deterioration.

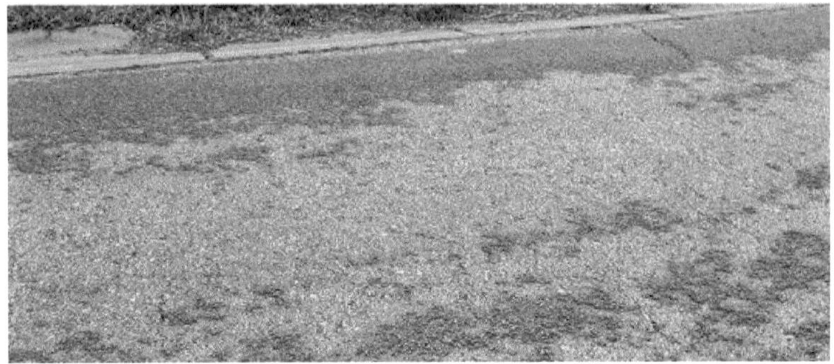

❖ Plumage :

Pluming is the gradual removal of chippings from a pavement, as shown in the figure below. Potential causes include underdosing of binder during surface dressing application, unfavorable atmospheric conditions such as low temperatures or rain during application, use of dirty chippings, insufficient compaction, spreading of unsuitable binder and too rapid a return to traffic. This deterioration is often observed in damp or shaded areas, where an overdose of binder may be necessary to reinforce the pavement's strength.

❖ Stripping :

Degradation of the mastic (binder and fines) around the aggregates of a wearing course, as shown in the figure below. Potential causes of this degradation include binder ageing, de-icing salt action, cleanliness of aggregates or sand, asphalt temperature at time of laying higher than specified, compaction failure (e.g. laying at lower temperatures).

Figure 42uncoating of asphalt pavement[24]

VII.1.4 Les Remontées :

❖ Penetrant testing

The condition of a rendering characterized by the rise of binder in slabs covering all or part of the aggregates, as illustrated in the figure below. Potential causes of this deterioration include overdosage of bitumen on partial emulsion applications or renderings, or the embedding of aggregates in a bituminous base that is too "soft" or too "greasy" (asphalt too rich in mastic).

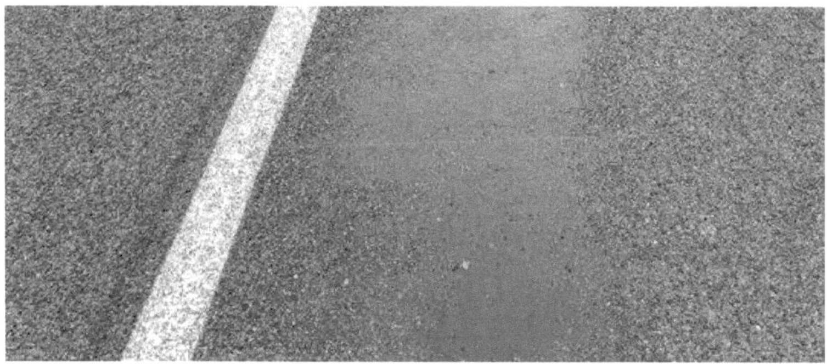

Figure 43Dye penetrant testing on asphalt pavement[25]

VII.2 Using fracture mechanics to study crack propagation in bituminous materials :

A number of researchers have explored the cracking behavior of bituminous materials, applying the principles of fracture mechanics. The following are some examples of crack propagation tests on bituminous materials.

VII.2.1 3-point bending test (SENB) :

The three-point bending test, also known as the Single Edge Notched Beam (SENB) test, represents an essential method for stressing a specimen in bending resting on two supports, with a load applied at equal distance from the two support points. Several crucial factors justify the use of this test.

Firstly, the size of the beam used in the SENB test is decisive, as it provides a substantial ligament, i.e. a significant zone of crack propagation. This extended ligament is essential for obtaining accurate data on the resistance of materials to cracking.

Secondly, another crucial aspect is the ability of the SENB test to induce mixed-mode failure. The basic configuration of this test can be easily adapted to test materials under mixed-mode conditions (Mode I and Mode II) simply by adjusting the initial notch located on the beam centerline. This capability is of particular importance in the analysis of bituminous pavements. Indeed, in this context, critical loads often result from a combination of thermal stresses (tension) and traffic-induced stresses (bending and shear stresses).

Consequently, the ability of the SENB test to characterize mixed-mode failure is particularly relevant to pavement studies and should be explored in greater detail in future research.

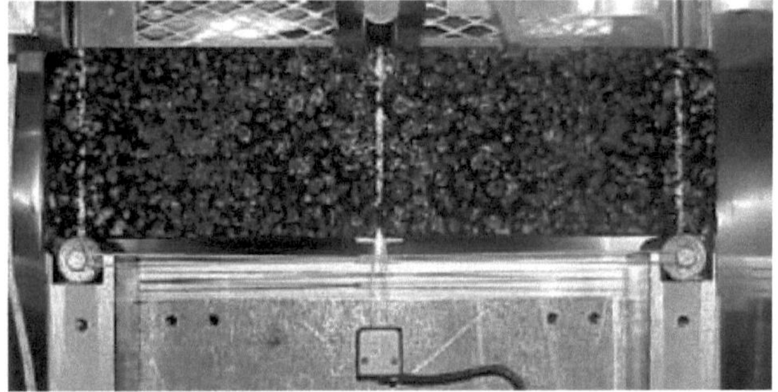

Figure 44 :Configuration of a 3-point bending test on asphalt mix[26]

VII.2.2 4-point bending test (FBNFT) :

The four-point bending test, known by its acronym FBNFT (Four Points Bending Notched Fracture Test), is a method for stressing a specimen in bending resting on two supports, with a load applied at two points symmetrical with respect to the midpoint between these two supports. Like the Three-Point Notched Fracture Test (SENB), the Four-Point Notched Fracture Test creates a significant crack propagation zone and offers the possibility of inducing mixed-mode fracture.

The major distinction between the four-point and three-point bending tests is that, in the case of the former, there is a constant moment between the two upper supports. This feature promotes more stable, controlled crack propagation throughout the test.

It should be emphasized that this increased crack stability can provide more reliable data when analyzing the cracking and fracture properties of materials. In addition, the ability to induce mixed-mode fracture remains an essential aspect of the test, making it a versatile method for characterizing the behavior of materials under complex bending stresses.

In addition, the FBNFT test also offers the possibility of studying the effect of different test parameters, such as applied load, specimen geometry, loading speed, etc., on crack propagation and material fracture toughness. This in-depth analytical capability enables us to gain a better understanding of material fracture mechanisms, and to guide the development of stronger, more durable materials in various fields of application.

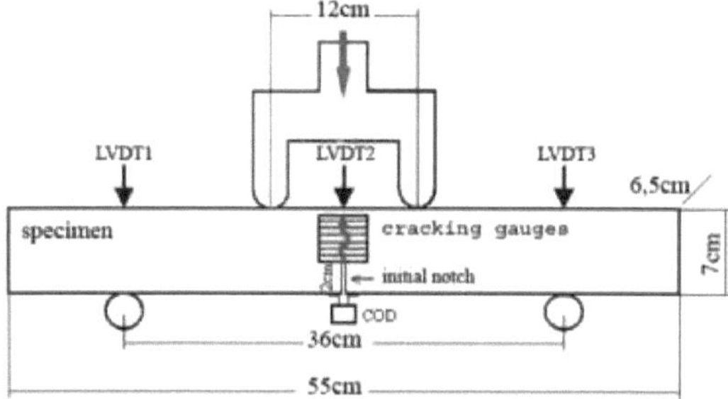

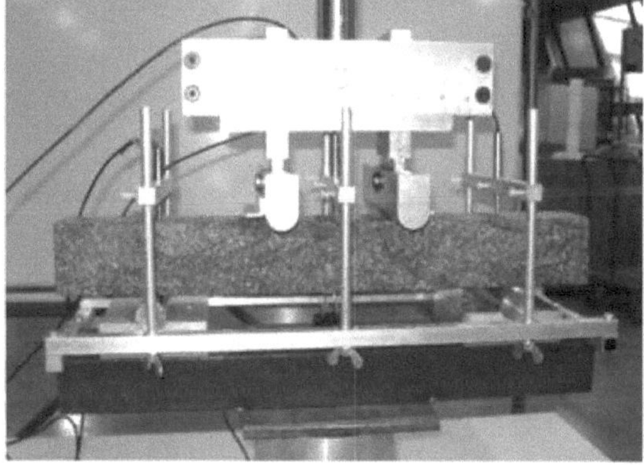

Figure 45:4-point bending test on a notched specimen from ENTPE[27]

VII.2.3 SCB test

The SCB test, or Semi-Circular Bending Test, is a test method used to assess the resistance to crack propagation of materials, particularly composite and bituminous materials. This test is particularly common in asphalt pavements.

In the SCB test, a semicircular specimen is first notched on one side to create an initial crack. This crack is often precisely shaped to ensure reproducible cracking conditions. The specimen is then subjected to a bending load applied to two bearing points located on opposite sides of the crack. This load configuration causes the specimen to bend and the crack to propagate through the material.

During the SCB test, the applied force and resulting deformation are measured to characterize the crack propagation resistance of the material under test. The data obtained is used to determine fracture toughness parameters such as crack propagation resistance and fracture energy. These parameters are essential for assessing material performance and designing crack-resistant structures. The table below summarizes the key elements of each SCB test standard. Each standard specifies different specimen configurations, such as notch length and thickness, required to conduct the test.

In summary, the SCB test is an important test method used to assess resistance to crack propagation in materials, particularly in asphalt mixes. It characterizes the fracture toughness properties of the material, providing valuable information for structural design and optimization.

Table 16Summary of key elements of each SCB test standard[28].

Standard	EN 12697-44:2010	AASHTO TP 105-13	ASTM D8044-16	AASHTO TP 124-18
Proposal year	2010	2013	2016	2018
Aim of the trial	Assessing the potential for crack propagation	Determine breaking energy (G), toughness (K) and stiffness (S) for low-temperature design in the mechanistic design guide Guide to mechanistic and empirical pavement design	Assessing the resistance to cracking of asphalt mixes at intermediate temperatures	Evaluate the breaking strength properties of asphalt mixes at temperatures as part of the mix approval process. mixture approval process
Test temperature	Below zero	Below the limit of the performance grade (PG) of the of binder used + 22 °C	5-35 °C	25 °C
Indicator	Tensile strength/ Fracture toughness	G, K, S	Critical deformation energy J-integral	Flexibility index *FI*
Sample diameter/ length of wing	150/10	150/15	150/25, 32, 38	150/15
Sample thickness (mm)	50 ± 3	24.7 ± 2	Laboratory sample: 57mm, pavement cores: minimum pavement layer	Laboratory sample: 50mm. pavement cores: minimum 25 mm

			thickness of 38mm.	
Loading rate	5 mm/min	0.0005 mm/s (0.03 mm/min)	0.5 mm/min	50 mm/min

VIII.　Study of asphalt cracking in different road sections using electrical resistivity tomography.

Based on the above, continuous exposure of asphalt pavements to seasonal weather variations associated with repeated vehicle loads and water infiltration through cracks, can result in weakened and saturated pavement structures, thus reducing the service life of asphalt pavements. [29]. In addition, delays in pavement renovation encourage moisture infiltration, which alters the internal structure of asphalt pavements and reduces their load-bearing capacity [30]. This in turn accelerates pavement deterioration, inevitably leading to higher repair costs, which can put a strain on a state's transport department budget.

To this end, it is essential to understand the dynamics of moisture and water circulation in the pavement support soil following the winter season, a major factor contributing to damage and cracking in asphalt pavements. This requires the application of a non-invasive method capable of providing on-site monitoring of cracking dynamics in asphalt pavements.

Orlando et al.[31] conducted an evaluation of various geophysical methods for diagnosing a rigid airport pavement. They used electromagnetic (EM) and georadar (GPR) techniques to generate high-resolution images of the pavement. In addition, electrical resistivity tomography (ERT) was used to definitively identify areas of anomaly. In addition, a seismic tomographic study was carried out to recover the mechanical properties of the pavement, including both P- and S-wave data, enabling the determination of elastic constants, including Poisson's ratio. Alsharahi et al. [32] used a combination of Georadar survey (GPR) and finite element simulation in different time domains (FDTD) to assess and identify the factors responsible for road collapse in northern Morocco. Chambers et al. [33] studied the internal moisture dynamics of a railway embankment using 2D and 3D resistivity measurements. Using 2D sections and 3D tomograms, they were able to track the development of seasonal moisture fronts with high spatial accuracy. They assessed moisture distributions on the sides, top and base of the embankment. Haryati and Alicia [34] studied subsurface conditions in damaged and undamaged pavement sections using electrical resistivity measurements under real field conditions. The electrical resistivity of damaged and undamaged pavement surfaces was measured and analyzed, focusing specifically on three types of defects: craze-like cracks in the bus parking area, ruts and potholes along the access road, and transverse cracks in the car parking area. The results of this study indicate variations in electrical resistivity values across the different defect types. Another study by Neyamadpour [35] used 2D electrical resistivity imaging using a Wenner-Schlumberger configuration to examine cracks on a road near the city of Masjed-Soleiman in Iran. This approach delineates the vertical extension of existing cracks in road structures. The inversion results revealed 17 distinct cracks, with depths ranging from 0.5 to 5.5 meters. Furthermore, in a study by Jackson et al. [36]2D electrical resistivity imaging was used to monitor the evolution of moisture distribution in a road embankment after pavement construction. This observation revealed an accumulation of moisture in the lower part of the embankment preceding a slope failure event. Another study by Rasul et al. [37] analyzed moisture in a cross-section of the E18 freeway in Sweden over one year using in situ electrical resistivity tomography (ERT). The ERT measuring line pre-installed under the asphalt surface layer of the road showed a high resistivity variation as a function of weather conditions, water flow and surface activities. Diallo et al. [38] conducted a study in Abu Dhabi, combining electrical resistivity tomography (ERT) and multichannel surface wave analysis (MASW) to characterize a road construction site and assess its infrastructure. This cost-effective approach integrated geophysical methods and geotechnical testing, providing a comprehensive, lateral characterization of subsurface materials. Nobahar et al. [39] investigated slope failures in highway embankments in Mississippi, constructed with highly shrinkable Yazoo clay, resulting from geotechnical, climatic and environmental factors. This poses maintenance problems for the Mississippi Department of Transportation. Various approaches, including electrical resistivity imaging (ERI) and finite element modeling (FEM), were explored. Drone and ERI imagery were used to locate problem areas in four failing embankments. The results of this study provide crucial data for the preventive assessment of embankment collapse, improving understanding of failure mechanisms, identifying contributing parameters, informing decision-making and selecting stabilization techniques, thereby enhancing the maintenance and sustainability of transport infrastructures.

Building on previous studies, this research used a non-destructive method called electrical resistivity tomography (ERT), which maps the spatial distribution of electrical soil properties beneath road surfaces. ERT is characterized by its low cost, ease of use and, above all, non-destructiveness [40]. It is also particularly well suited to shallow investigations [41] and promising for its ability to detect lithological variations [42]. In addition, it can also be used to visualize changes in soil moisture by applying appropriate petrophysical relationships that relate resistivity to saturation [43,44].

To this end, ERT is being applied to four distinct road sections, each showing different types of cracking and damage in the asphalt pavement, at different time intervals, before and during the winter season. The results of the ERT investigations will be supplemented by visual assessments of asphalt pavement deterioration and core sampling.

Consequently, the main objective of this study is to investigate the relationship between soil electrical resistivity and the specific types of cracking observed in bituminous pavements. In addition, the study aims to assess the impact of moisture dynamics and water circulation in the soil supporting the pavement, particularly during the winter season, in order to gain a deeper understanding of the factors influencing road durability, particularly in the Moroccan context. The results of this research have the potential to improve road maintenance and construction practices, thereby promoting the development of more resilient and sustainable infrastructures.

VIII.1 Visual survey of damage on different road sections:

VIII.1.1Route Régionale 707 between Elhajeb and Ifrane :

VIII.1.1.1 Location of road section to be visually surveyed :

The section of road surveyed extends over 36 kilometers along RR707 between Elhajeb and Ifrane, as shown in the figure above. Its starting point, PK 0 for the survey, is in Elhajeb, while its end point is in Ifrane. This section has an AADT (2021 traffic census) of 3008 veh/d, with a percentage of heavy goods vehicles of 9.28% and a traffic growth rate of 4%, according to the 2021 census manual drawn up by the Road Directorate.

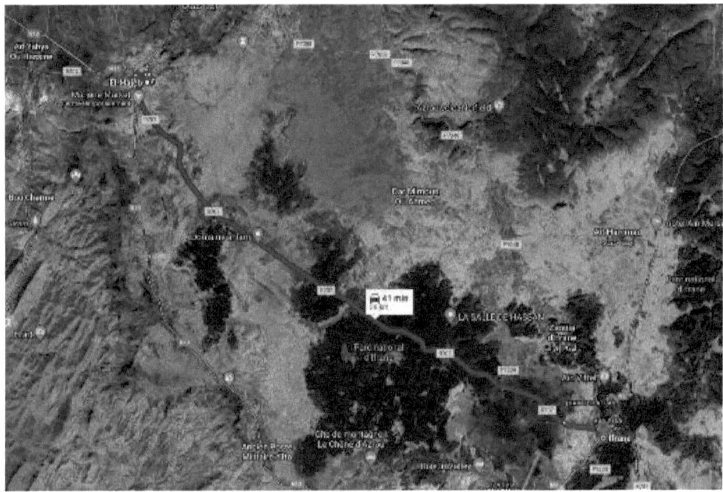

Figure 46Location of the section of road covered by the visual survey

VIII.1.1.2 Visual survey of damage on the section of road to be visually surveyed :

A visual inspection of the roadway revealed the following:

- ✓ The wearing course of the road is asphalt and marked by the presence of cracks in places (longitudinal cracking - beginning of crazing - crazing).
- ✓ The MS shoulders are slightly eroded and uneven in relation to the roadway.

We note that the roadway has recently undergone maintenance work, extending from KP 15 to KP 36, where it is in good condition.

All damage is listed in the table below:

Table 17Damage to road section RR 707

Section		Rive	Illustration	Comment
From KP	At KP			
0+000	0+700	D+G	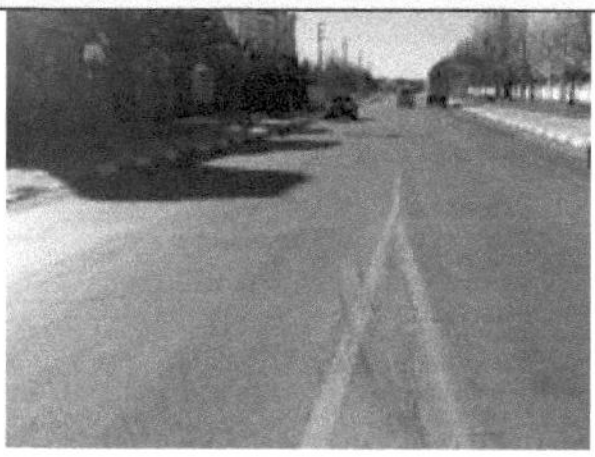	The damage observed consists of crazing, longitudinal and transverse cracks on both sides of the roadway.
1+700	1+800	D+G		The damage observed is of the crazing type along the centreline of the road.
2+300	2+400	D+G	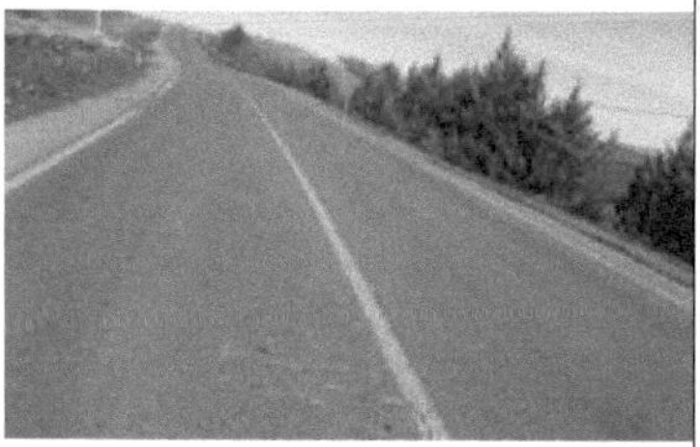	The damage observed is of the crazing type along the centreline of the road.
2+500	3+200	D+G	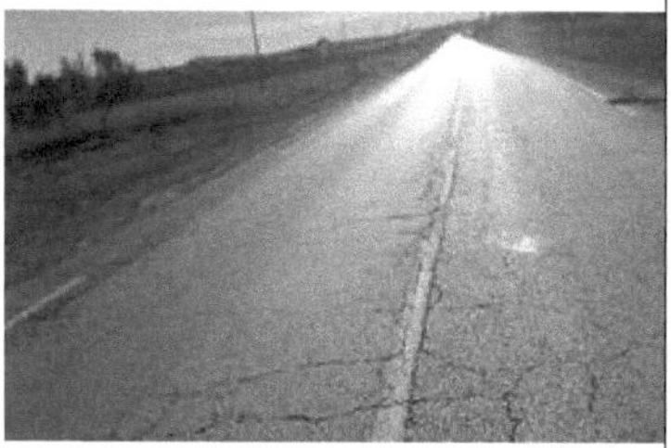	The damage observed is of the "faiençage" type, on both sides of the roadway.

<table>
<tr><th colspan="2">Section</th><th>Riv
e</th><th>Illustration</th><th rowspan="2">Comment</th></tr>
<tr><th>From
KP</th><th>At
KP</th><th></th><th></th></tr>
<tr><td>3+20
0</td><td>3+60
0</td><td>D</td><td> 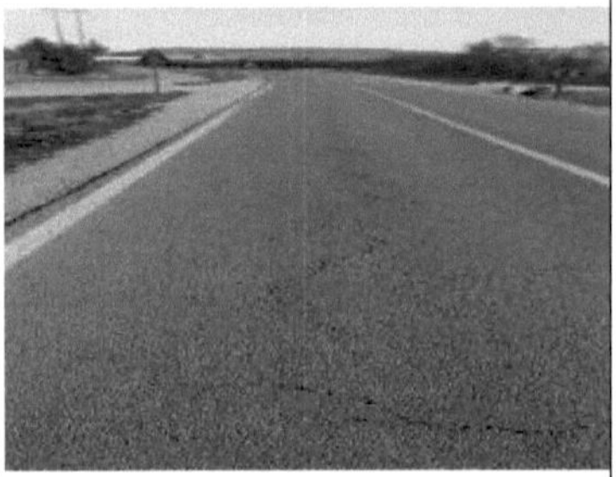</td><td>The damage observed is of the faience type, on the right bank of the roadway.</td></tr>
<tr><td>3+70
0</td><td>3+90
0</td><td>D+
G</td><td> 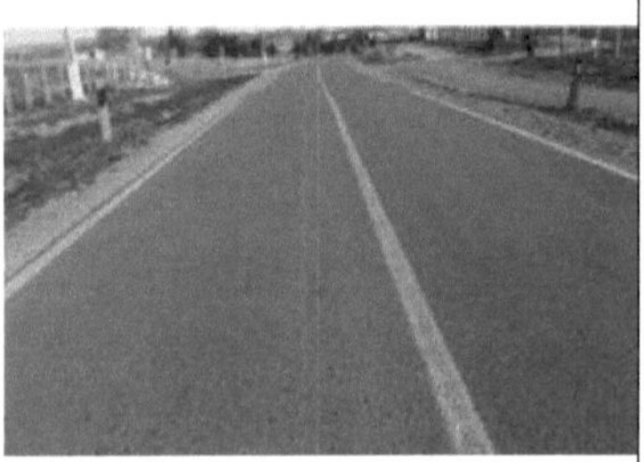</td><td>The damage observed is of the "faiençage" type, on both sides of the roadway.</td></tr>
<tr><td>4+20
0</td><td>4+60
0</td><td>G</td><td> 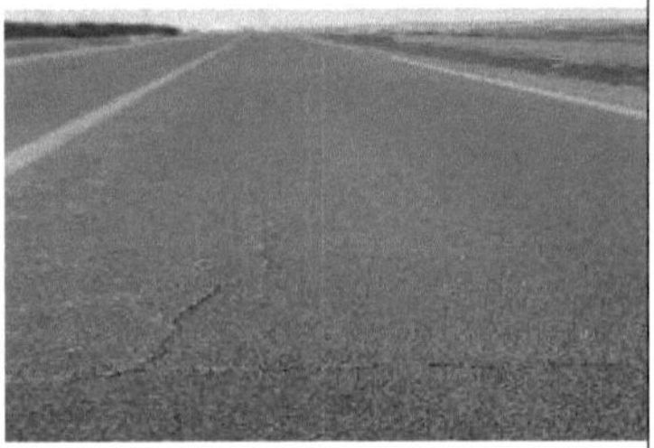</td><td>The damage observed consists of crazing, longitudinal and transverse cracks on the left bank of the roadway.</td></tr>
</table>

Section		Riv e	Illustration	Comment
From KP	**At KP**			
5+200	5+800	D+ G	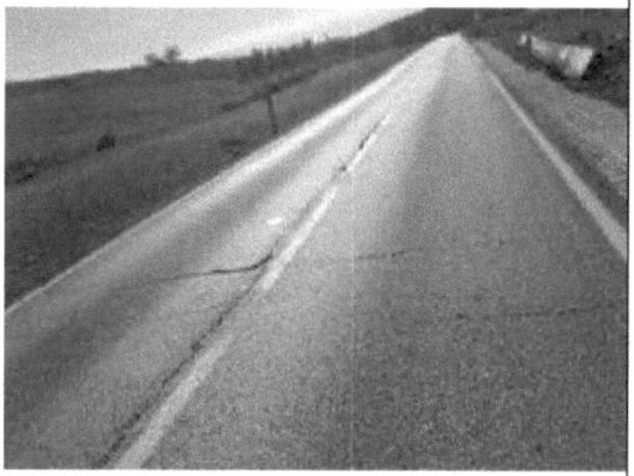	The damage observed consists of crazing, longitudinal cracks along the axis and transverse cracks on both sides of the roadway.
5+800	6+100	G	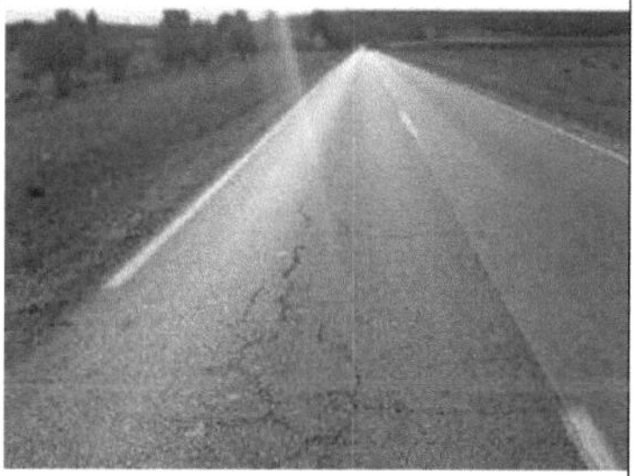	The damage observed consists of crazing on the left bank of the roadway.
6+100	6+800	D+ G	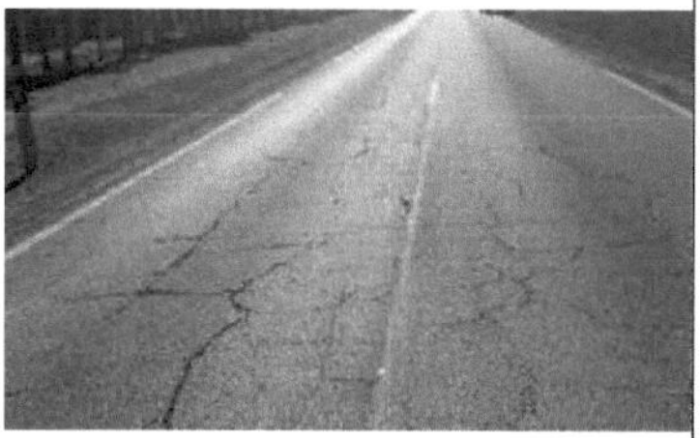	The damage observed consists of crazing, longitudinal and transverse cracks on both sides of the roadway.
7+200	7+700	G	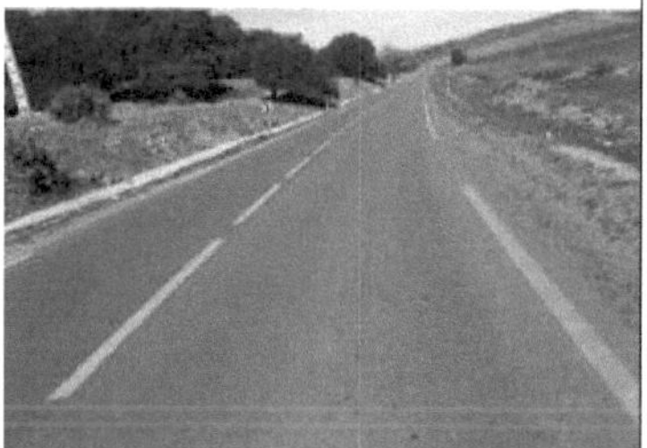	The damage observed is of the faience type, on the left bank of the roadway.
From KP	**At KP**			

Section		Riv e	Illustration	Comment
From KP	**At KP**			
7+80 0	7+90 0	D+ G	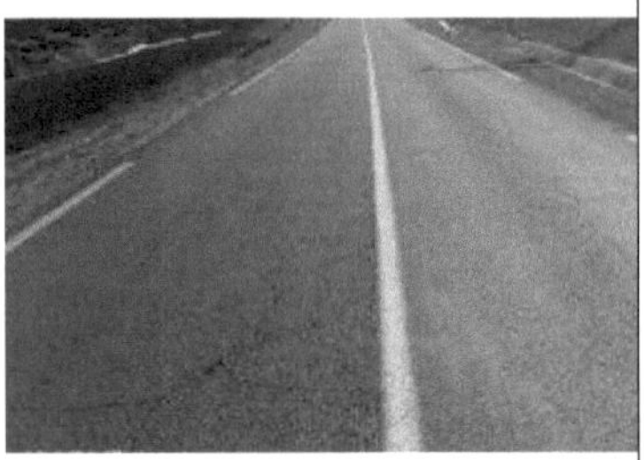	The damage observed is of the faience type, on both sides of the roadway.
8+70 0	8+80 0	D	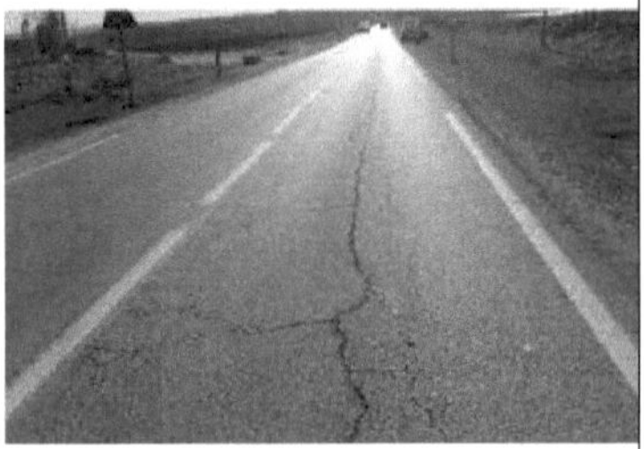	The damage observed consists of crazing and longitudinal cracking on the right-hand side of the roadway.
10+0 00	10+4 00	G	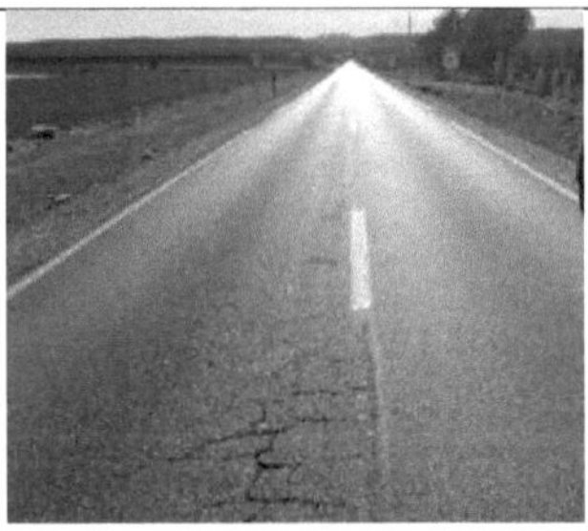	The damage observed is of the faience type, on the left bank of the roadway.
10+6 00	11+6 00	D+ G	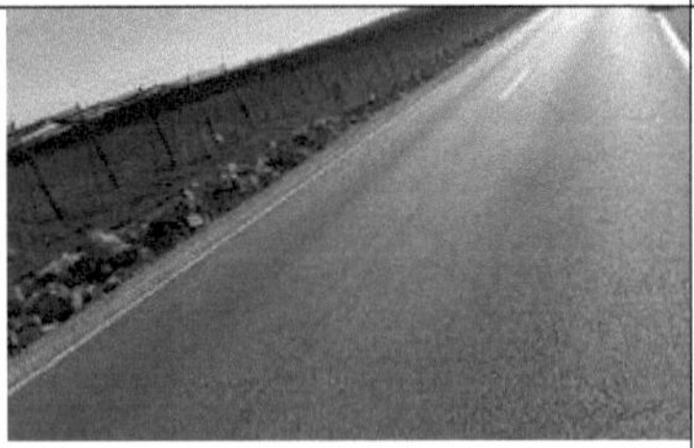	The damage observed is of the crazing type, less pronounced on both sides of the roadway.

Section		Rive	Illustration	Comment
From KP	**At KP**	**Riv e**		
12+9 00	13+2 00	D+ G	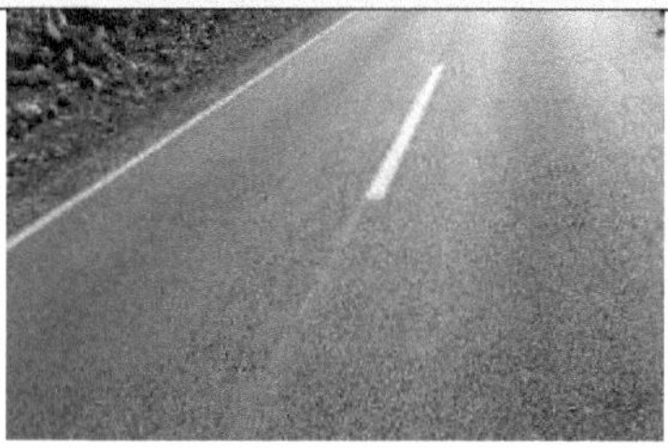	The damage observed is of the crazing type, less pronounced on both sides of the roadway.
13+2 00	13+4 00	G	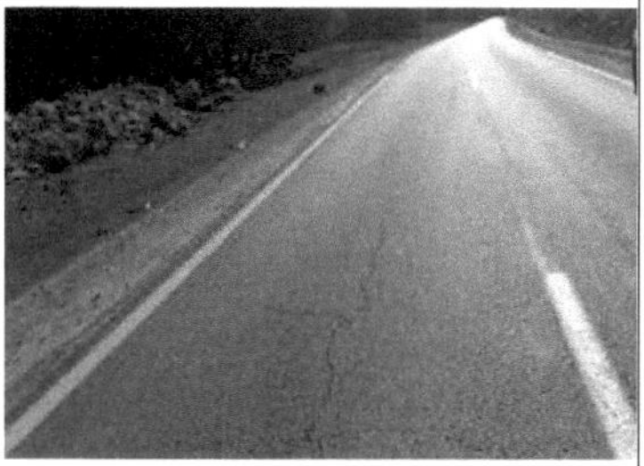	The damage observed consists of crazing and longitudinal cracking on the left bank of the roadway.
13+7 00	14+5 00	D+ G	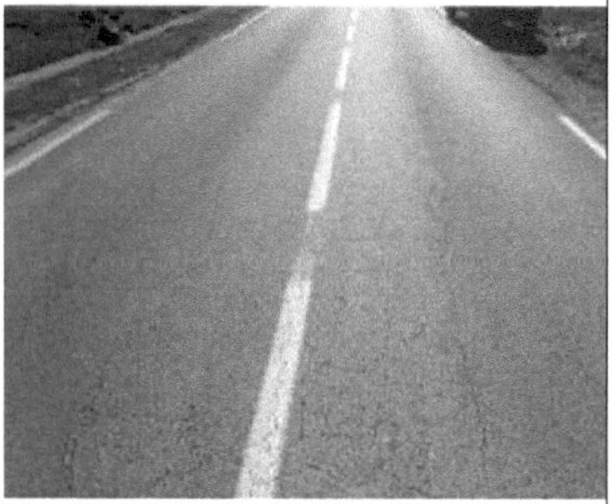	The damage observed is of the crazing type, less pronounced on both sides of the roadway.

(*) PK: Kilometre point; RD: Right bank; RG: Left bank

VIII.1.2 National road RN 13 between Aglmam Sidi Ali and Hjirt :

VIII.1.2.1 Location of the road section to be visually surveyed :

The section of road surveyed extends over 10 kilometers on the RN 13 between Aglmam Sidi Ali and Hjirt, as shown in the figure above. Its starting point, noted PK 0 for the survey, is at Aglmam Sidi Ali, while its end point is at Hjirt.

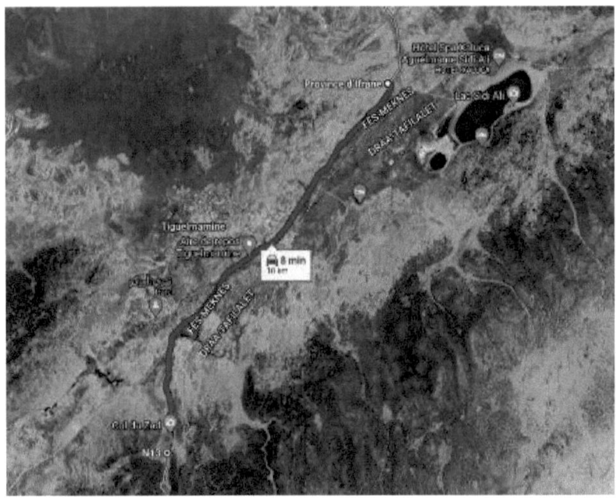

Figure 47Location of the section of road covered by the visual survey

VIII.1.2.2 Visual survey of damage on the section of road to be visually surveyed :

A visual inspection of the roadway revealed the following:

- ✓ The wearing course of the roadway is asphalt and marked by the presence of cracks in places (longitudinal cracking, transverse cracking and crazing).

- ✓ Slight deformation marked by subsidence in places.

- ✓ The MS shoulders are slightly eroded and uneven in relation to the roadway.

All damage is listed in the table below:

Table 18 Damage to the RN13 road section

Section		Rive	illustration	Comment
From KP	At KP	e		
0+000	0+200	G	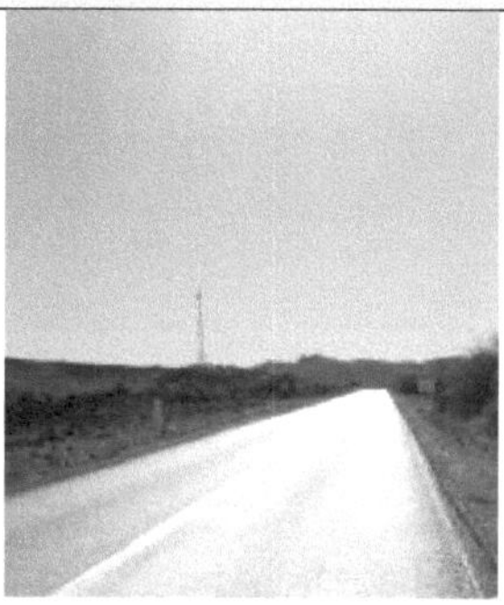	Damage observed includes crazing at the edge, longitudinal cracks
0+300	0+500	D+ G	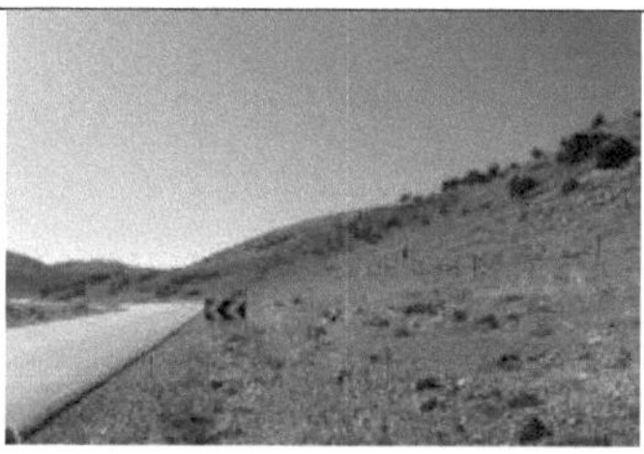	The MS shoulders are slightly eroded and uneven in relation to the roadway.
1+500	2+500	D+ G	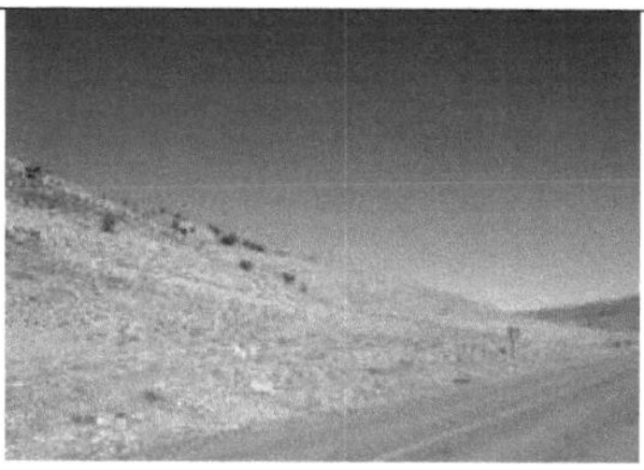	The MS shoulders are slightly eroded and uneven in relation to the roadway.
4+000	-	D+ G	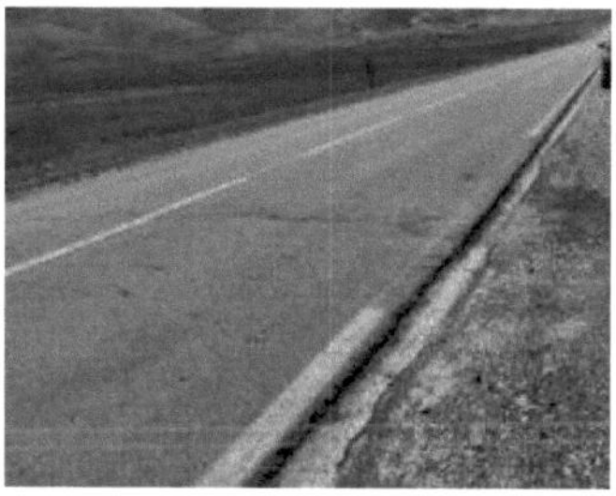	The MS shoulders are marked by slight erosion. Fissure-type transverse crack.

Section		Rive	illustration	Comment
From KP	At KP	e		
4+000	5+00 0	D+ G	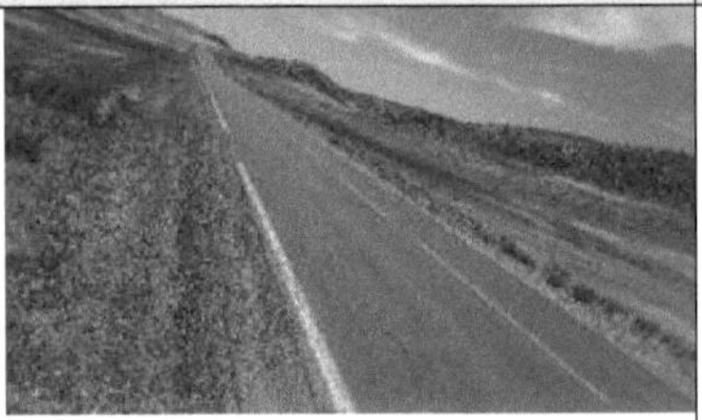	The MS shoulders are marked by slight erosion. Fissure-type transverse crack. Longitudinal crack at the edge
5+400	5+30 0	D+ G	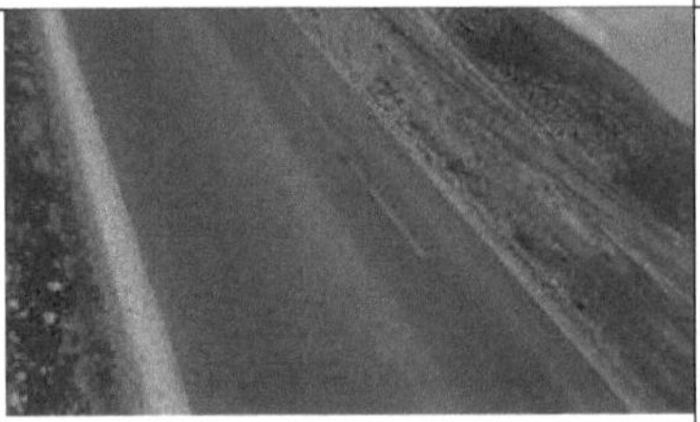	Longitudinal crack in the road axis
6+00	6+30 0	D+ G	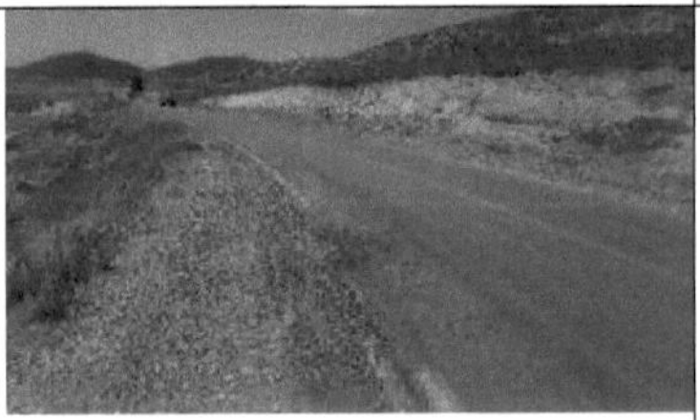	Bank subsidence and weakening
			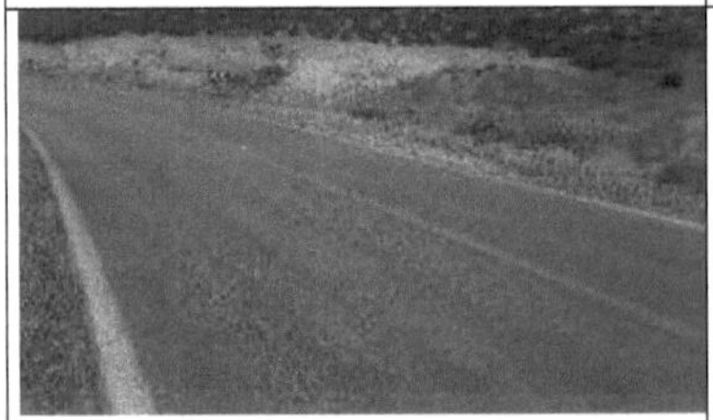	Fissure-type transverse crack.
7+000	8+00 0	D+ G	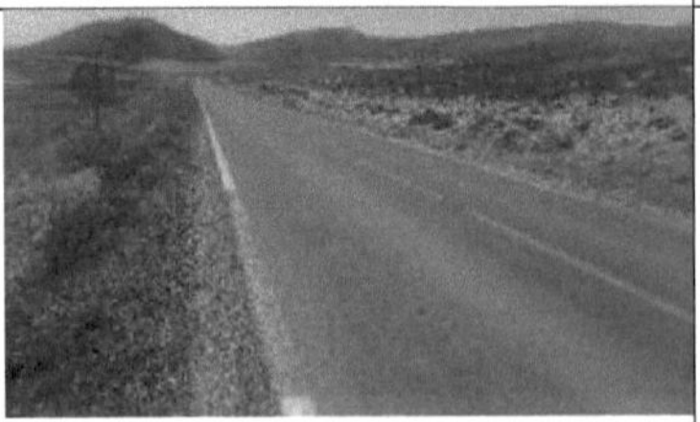	The MS shoulders are slightly eroded and uneven in relation to the roadway.

Section		Riv e	illustration	Comment
From KP	**At KP**			
8+800	-	D	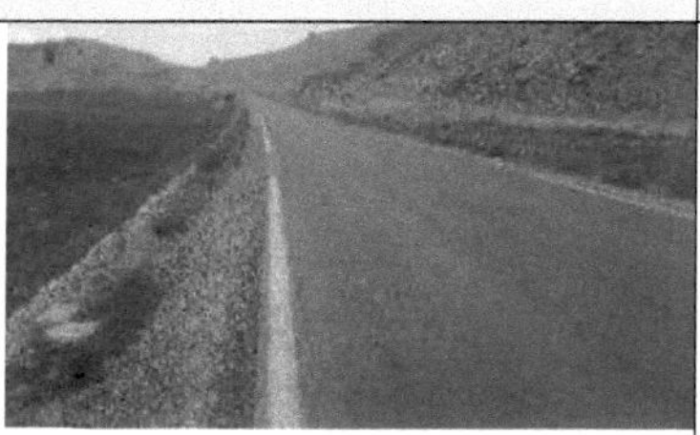	Right bank subsidence and longitudinal crack
9+100	9+20 0	D	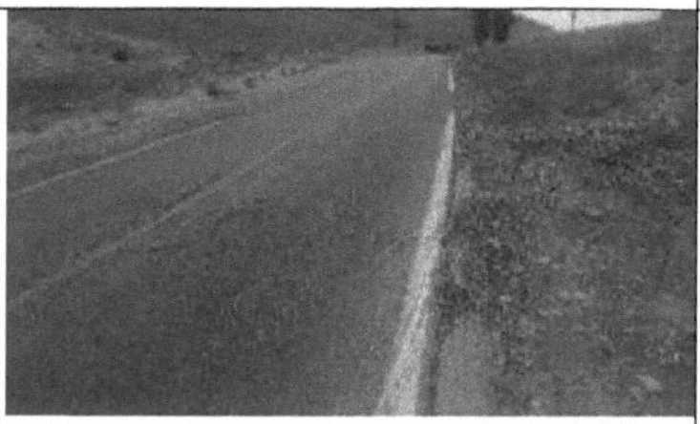	The MS shoulders are slightly eroded and uneven in relation to the roadway. Subsidence of the right bank and transverse cracking (beginning of crazing)

VIII.1.3 National road N°8 between Immouzzar and Ifrane :

VIII.1.3.1 Location of the road section to be visually surveyed :

The section of road surveyed extends over 21.7 km along the RN 8 between Immouzzar and Ifrane, as shown in the figure above. Its starting point, noted PK 0 for the survey, is in Immouzzar, while its end point is in Ifrane. This section has an AADT (2021 traffic census) of 7200 veh/d, with a percentage of heavy goods vehicles of 8.96% and a traffic growth rate of 4%, according to the 2021 census manual drawn up by the Road Directorate.

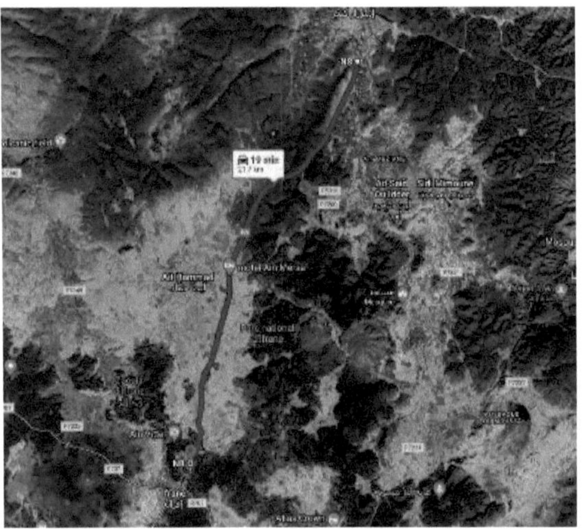

Figure 48Location of the section of road covered by the visual survey

VIII.1.3.2 Visual survey of damage on the section of road to be visually surveyed :

A visual inspection of the roadway revealed the following:

- ✓ The wearing course of the roadway is asphalt and marked by the presence of cracks in places (longitudinal cracking - beginning of crazing - crazing) and collapsed banks.

- ✓ The MS shoulders are slightly eroded and uneven in relation to the roadway.

All damage is listed in the table below:

Table 19 Damage to the RN 8 road section

Section		Illustration	Comment
From KP	At KP		
0+000	0+500		Right bank subsidence Faience Longitudinal crack Roadside erosion
0+750	1+000		Slight subsidence on right bank Beginning of crazing Roadside erosion
1+600	1+800		Longitudinal crack Beginning of crazing on right bank

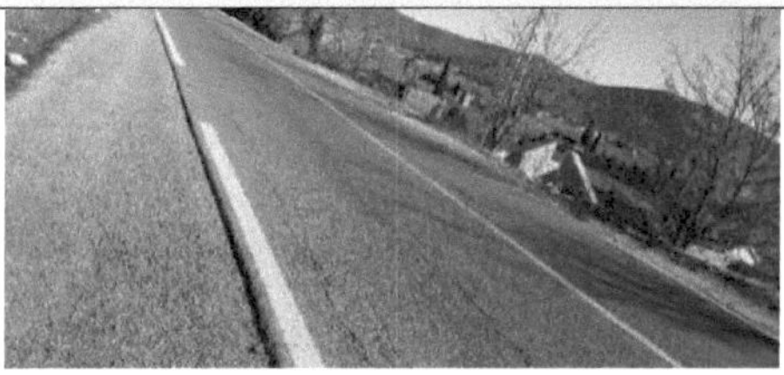

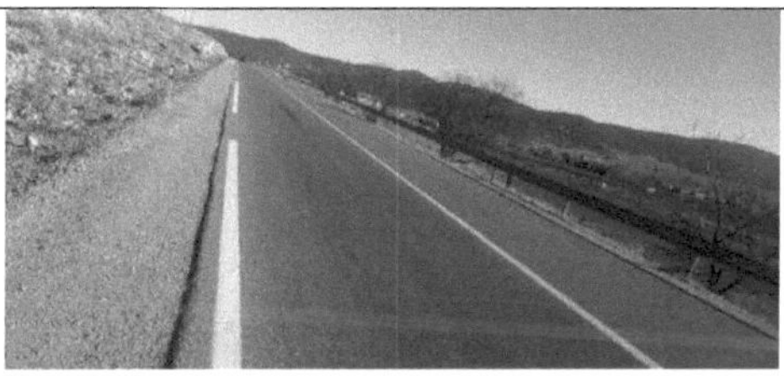

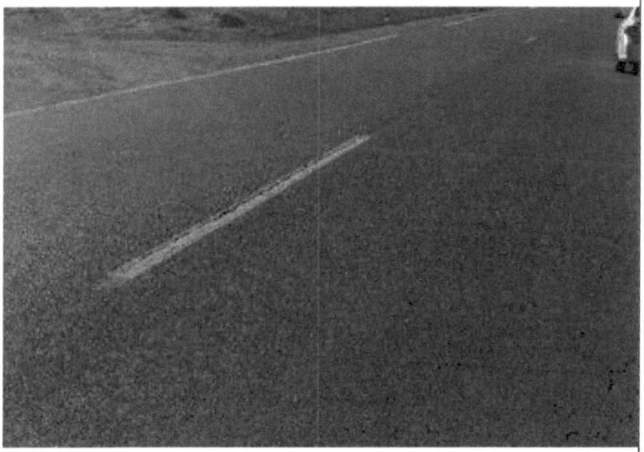

Section		Illustration	Comment
Fro m KP	At KP		
1+90 0	2+05 0	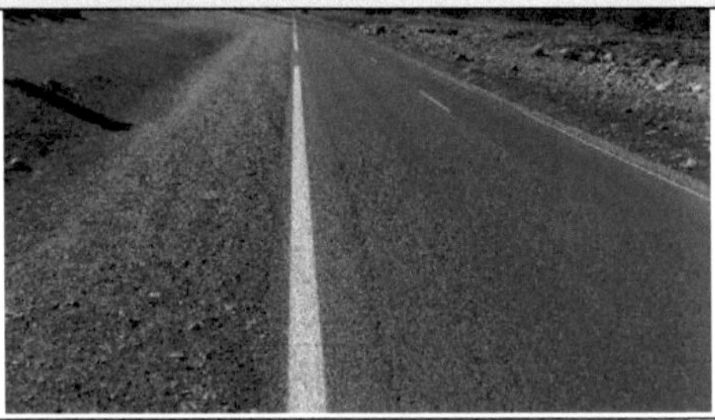	Longitudi nal crack. Beginning of crazing on left bank.
2+15 0	2+30 0		Slight longitudin al crack. Beginning of crazing on right bank. Embankm ent subsidenc e.
3+00 0	3+10 0	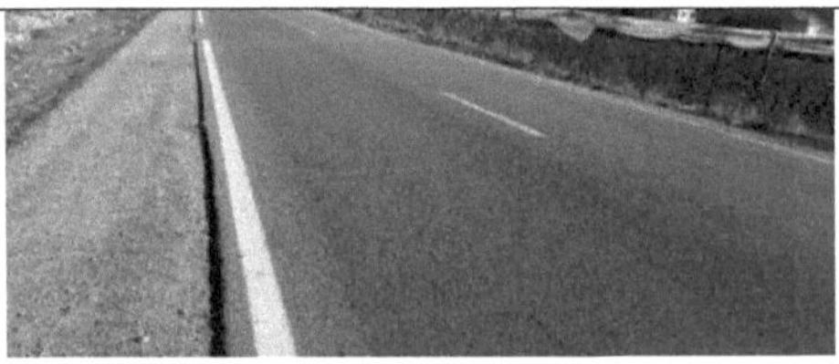	Slight longitudin al crack. Beginning of crazing on right bank. Embankm ent subsidenc e. Shoulder erosion.

Section		Illustration	Comment
Fro m KP	**At KP**		
3+90 0	4+15 0	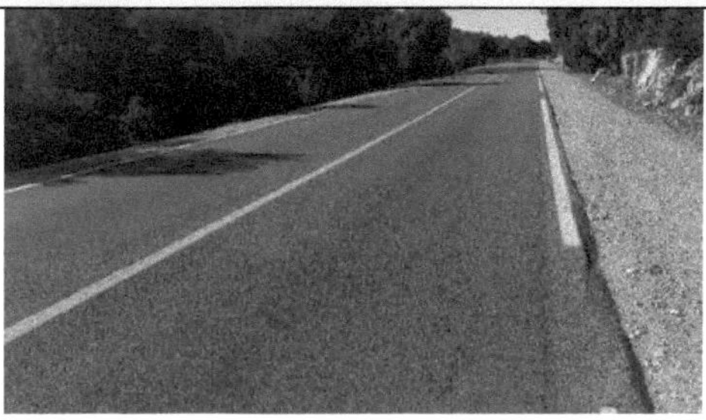	Longitudi nal crack Beginning of crazing on right bank
9+80 0	10+4 00	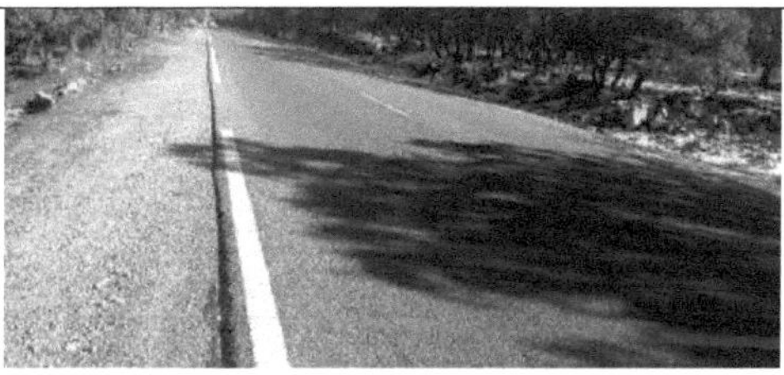	Slight subsidenc e on right bank Beginning of crazing Transvers e crack
10+6 00	11+1 00	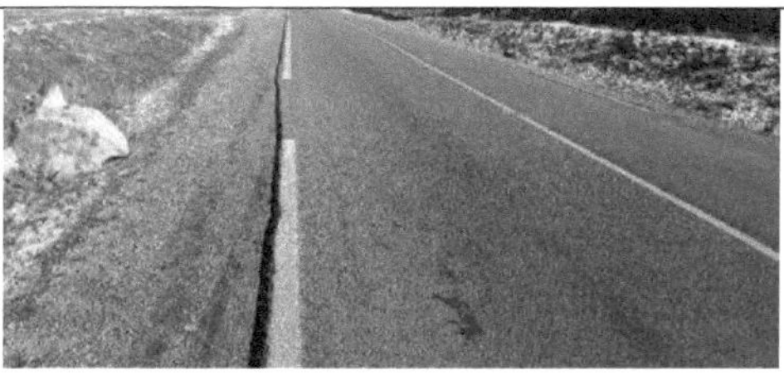	Slight subsidenc e on right bank Beginning of crazing Shoulder erosion.
11+2 00	11+2 00	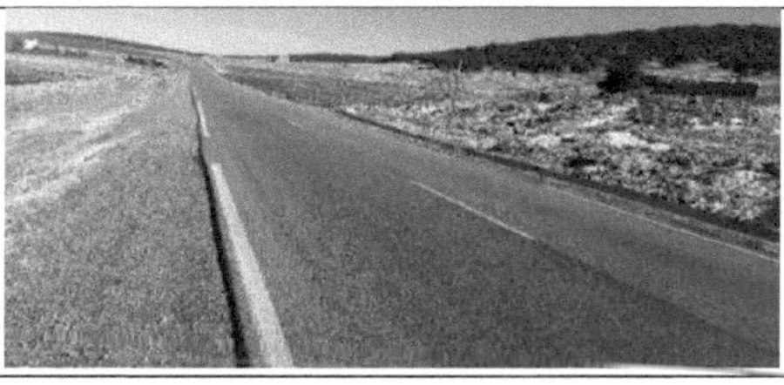	Crackling right bank Roadside erosion

Section		Illustration	Comment
Fro m KP	**At KP**		
17+0 00	17+2 50	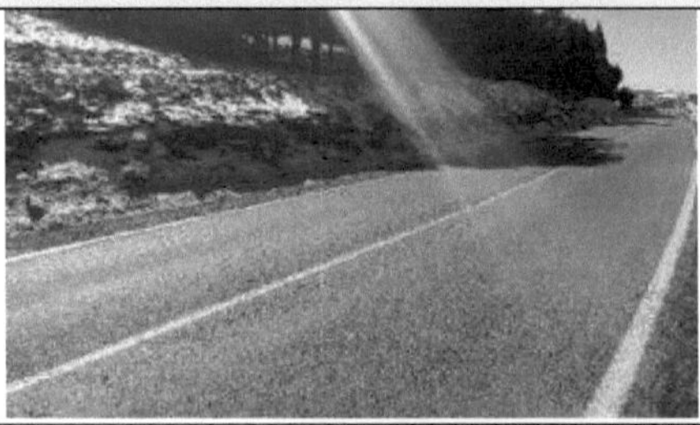	Faïençage axis of the roadway.
17+6 00	17+4 00	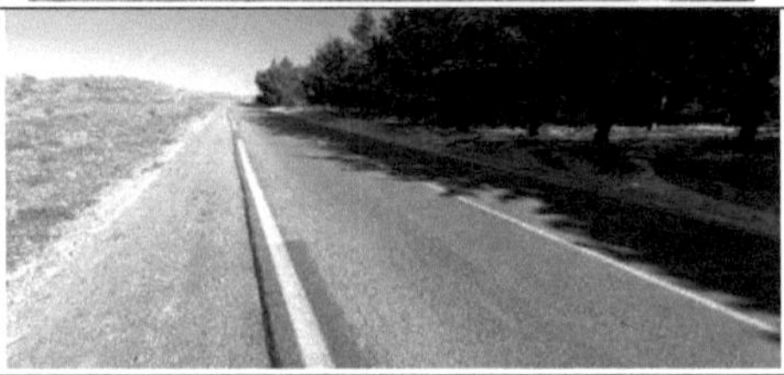	Crackling right bank
18+2 00	18+4 00	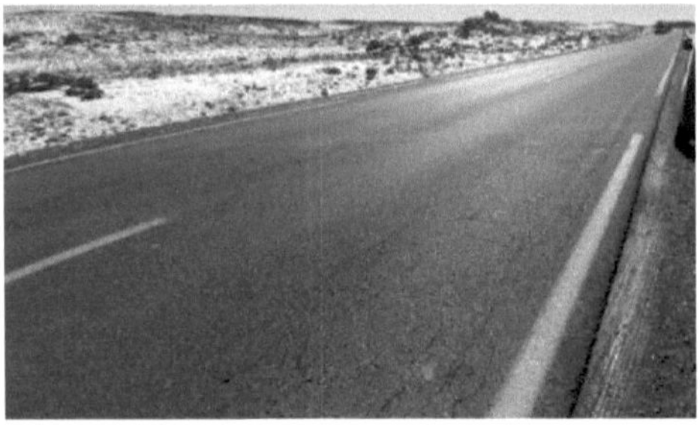	Crackling right bank
18+5 00	18+7 00	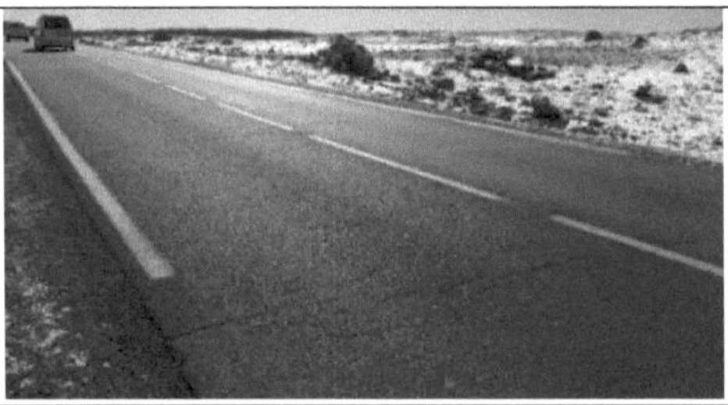	Transvers e crack Beginning of crazing

Section		Illustration	Comment
Fro m KP	**At KP**		
18+9 00	19+0 00	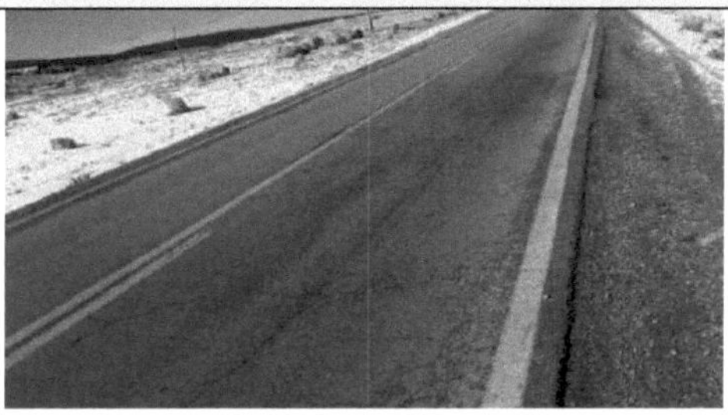	Right bank subsidenc e Faience
20+3 00	20+3 50	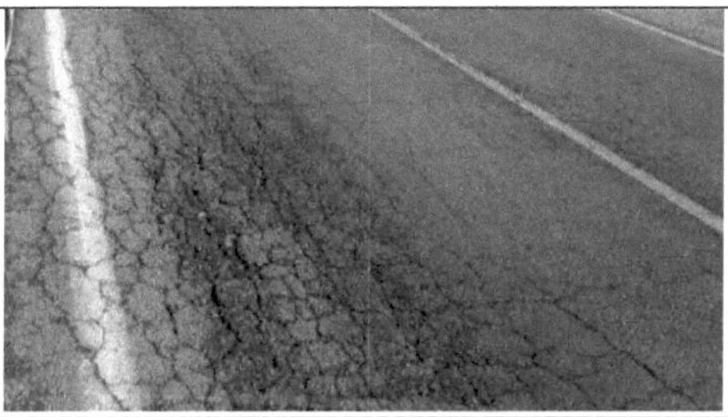	Right bank subsidenc e Faience

VIII.2 Location and description of road sections to be surveyed :

VIII.2.1 Road section N°1 :

The section of road is located 11 km northwest of the town of Ifrane, on the regional road RR707. Visual inspection of the road surface revealed signs of early longitudinal and transverse cracking, as shown in Figure 49. The soil supporting the road is composed of fractured limestone with clay joints, as indicated by the outcrop of the Figure 50.

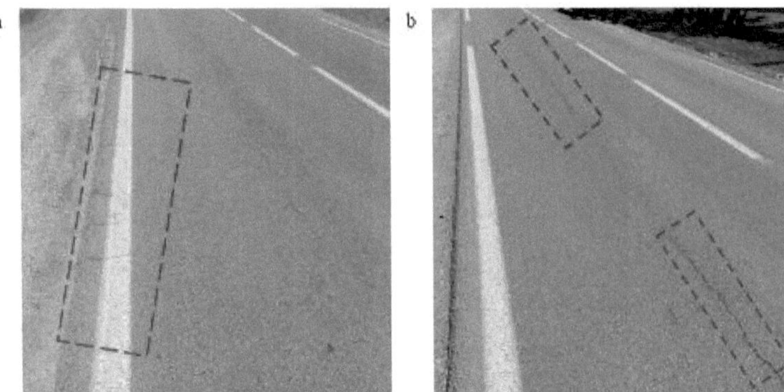

Figure 49(a) Transverse crack in asphalt pavement; (b) Longitudinal crack in asphalt pavement.

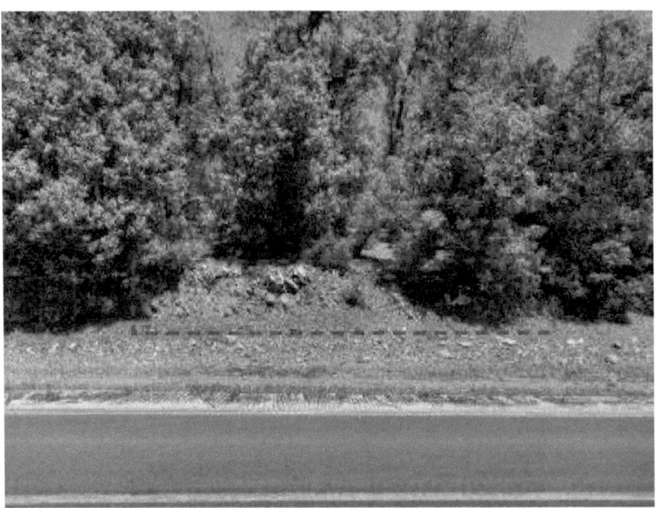

Figure 50:Fractured limestone outcrop with clay joints

VIII.2.2 Section Routière N°2 :

The road section is located 4 km south-east of the town of Ifrane, on the regional road RR707. Visual inspection of the road surface revealed the presence of advanced cracking, characterized by the presence of Raveling on the bituminous pavement and cracks along the road axis, with erosion of the bituminous pavement on the road edges, as shown in Figure 51. The supporting soil is composed of fractured limestone, as shown by the outcrop in Figure 52.

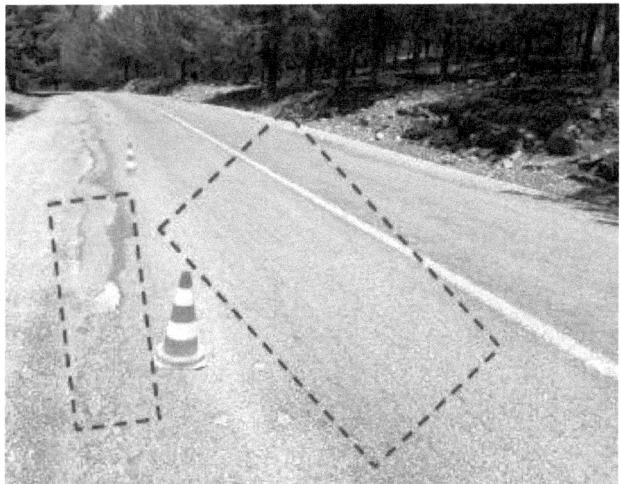

Figure 51:Visual inspection of pavement damage

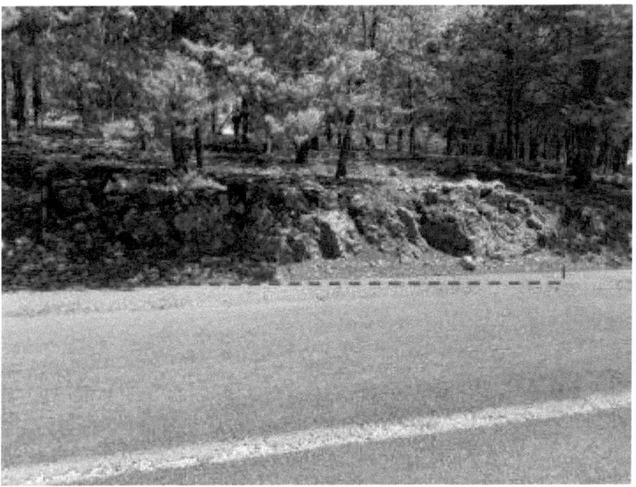

Figure 52Fractured limestone outcrop.

VIII.2.3 Road section N°3

The section of road is located 8 km south-east of the town of Azrou, on the RN13 national highway. Visual inspection of the road surface revealed the presence of advanced cracking along the road axis, with erosion of the bituminous pavement on the road edges, as shown in Figure 53. The soil supporting the road is composed of fractured limestone, as shown by the outcrop in Figure 54.

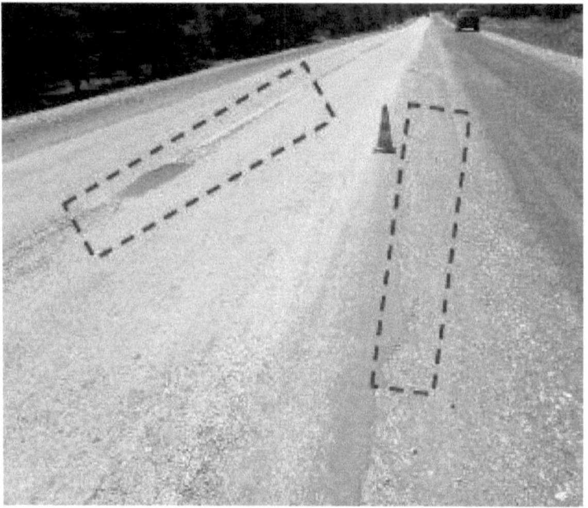

Figure 53:Visual inspection of pavement deterioration

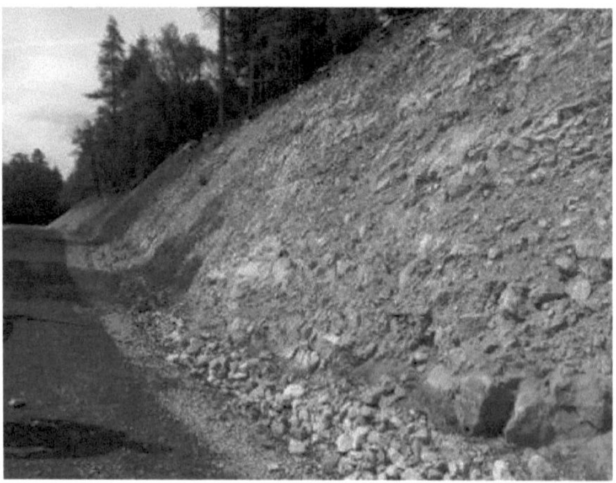

Figure 54Fractured limestone outcrop.

VIII.2.4Road section N°4

The section of road is located 23 km north of the town of Timahdite, on the RN13 national highway. Visual inspection of the road surface revealed the presence of advanced cracks perpendicular to the road axis, as shown in Figure 55. The soil supporting the road is composed of clayey silt, as shown by the excavation carried out with a backhoe, indicated in Figure 56.

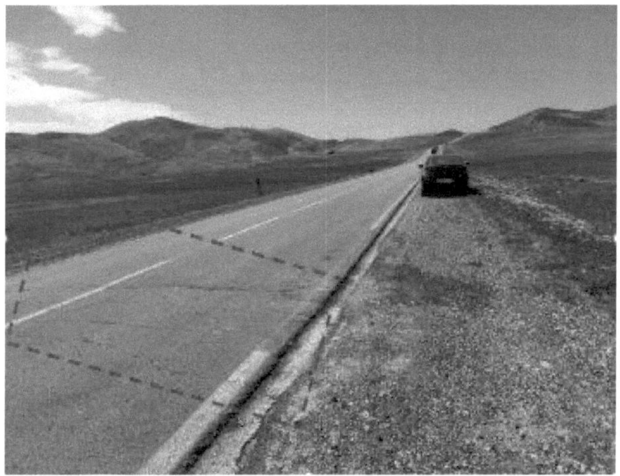

Figure 55Cracks perpendicular to the road axis on the pavement.

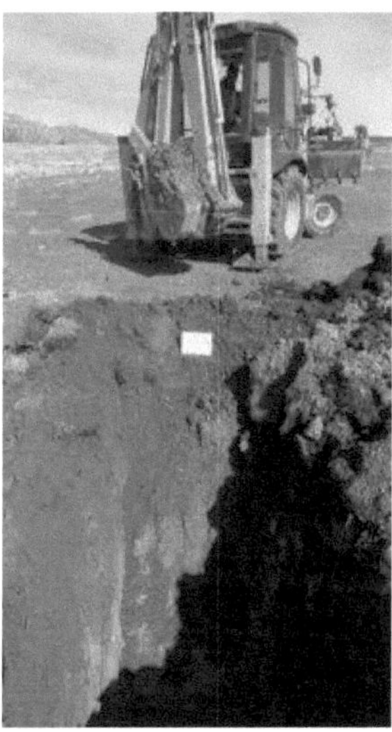

Figure 56Shovel hole revealing the presence of clayey silts

VIII.3 Materials and methodology :

Following visual inspection of the various types of cracks and damage observed on the bituminous pavements along the road sections, two geophysical campaigns will be carried out in November 2022, just before the start of the winter season, and another in February 2023, during the winter season. These campaigns will measure electrical resistivity in different road sections and at the same locations in the study areas.

The equipment used to measure electrical resistivity is ABEM's Terrameter LS with a multi-electrode system. This system consists of 32 electrodes nailed to the shoulders of the pavements studied, along the resistivity measurement line established according to the WENNER protocol, with a spacing of 5.0 meters between each electrode, as illustrated in Figure 57.

The principle of the WENNER protocol is to keep the current and potential electrodes at the same distance from each other. At each stage, a measurement is recorded, and the sum of all these measurements at this first inter-electrode spacing gives a profile of resistivity values. Next, the inter-electrode spacing is increased by a factor of n = 2, and a second line of measurements is taken. This process is repeated until the maximum electrode spacing is reached [22,45,46] as shown in Figure 58.

Electrical tomography profiles were interpreted using RES2DINV resistivity and induced polarization interpretation software. These investigations were combined with visual surveys of the state of deterioration of the asphalt pavements and core drilling, the Figure 59 summarizes the methodology used in this research.

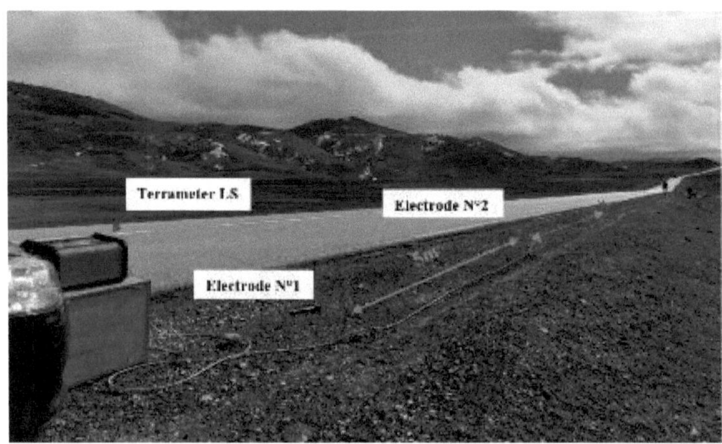

Figure 57 :Electrical resistivity measurement with Terrameter LS

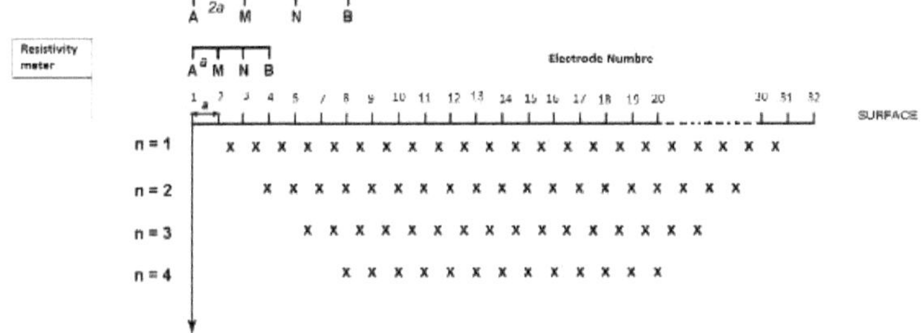

Figure 58:Wenner protocol for 2D electrical imaging data acquisition

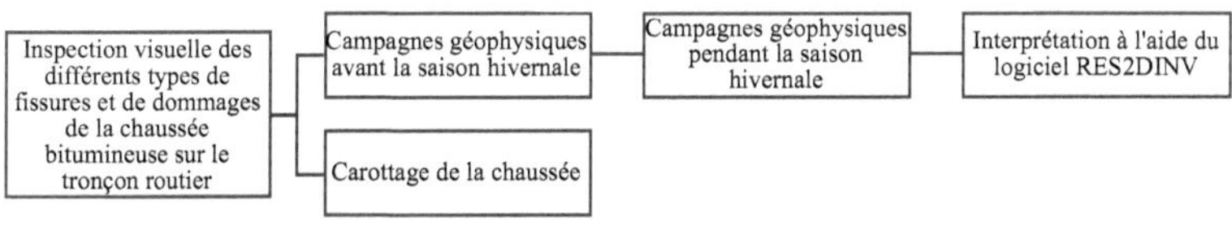

Figure 59:The methodology used in this research.

VIII.4 Geophysical survey results:

Two geophysical campaigns will be carried out in November 2022, just before the start of the winter season, and another in February 2023, during the winter season. These campaigns will measure electrical resistivity in different road sections and at the same locations in the study areas. The measurement lines extend over a total distance of 160 metres.

VIII.4.1 Road section N°1 :

The pseudosection presents the results of 2D electrical resistivity measurements performed on a bituminous pavement showing premature longitudinal and transverse cracking, as illustrated in the Figure 60.

The cracks appear at the beginning of the line over a length of 80 metres. Electrical resistivity values under the defective pavement zone range from 50 to 95 ohms.meter. In contrast, resistivity values in the non-defective area are higher, ranging from 150 to 360 ohms.meter. More precisely, in the Figure 60 (b), a decrease in electrical resistivity is observed over a distance of 20 meters, between points 80 and 110 meters, with resistivity values ranging from 50 to 70 ohms.meter, shown in blue. Pre-winter resistivity values range from 150 to 300 ohms.meter, as shown in green on the profile in Figure 60 (a).

In addition, the results of pavement coring, revealing the presence of a 16 cm thick layer of bituminous material resting on a gravel layer, as illustrated in Figure 61.

Examination of the visual inspection and the results obtained reveals a number of important points. In particular, a clear formation discontinuity on the surface suggests the presence of a contact anomaly between two distinct soil types: a conductive soil (with resistivity values between 50 and 90 ohms.meter) at the start of the profile and a resistant soil (with resistivity values between 150 and 300 ohms.meter), mainly attributed to fractured limestone. In addition, the conductive zone extends during the winter season, mainly due to rainwater infiltration and the specific characteristics of the pavement support soil, composed of fractured limestone with clayey joints that allow water to circulate. This environment is conducive to the creation of a zone liable to degrade the asphalt pavement. Premature cracking in the current state of the pavement can be attributed to the thickness of the asphalt layer, which offers a certain resistance to deterioration. Conversely, undamaged areas of pavement are associated with more resistant limestone formations.

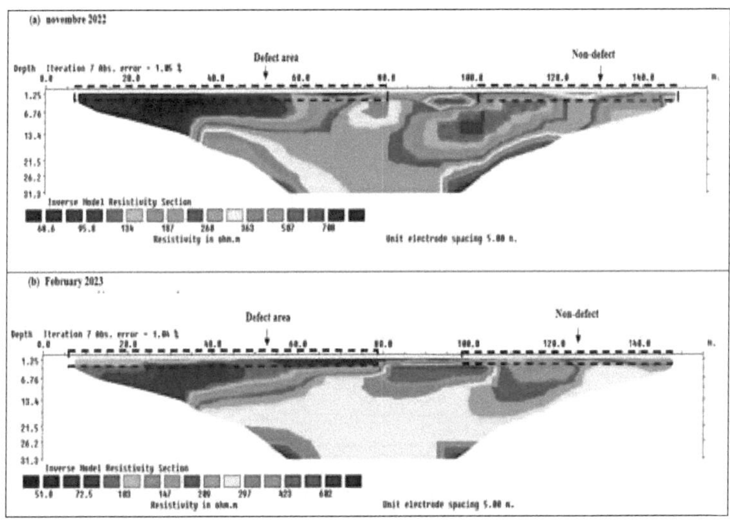

Figure 60(a) 2D resistivity image before the winter season (b) 2D resistivity image during the winter season

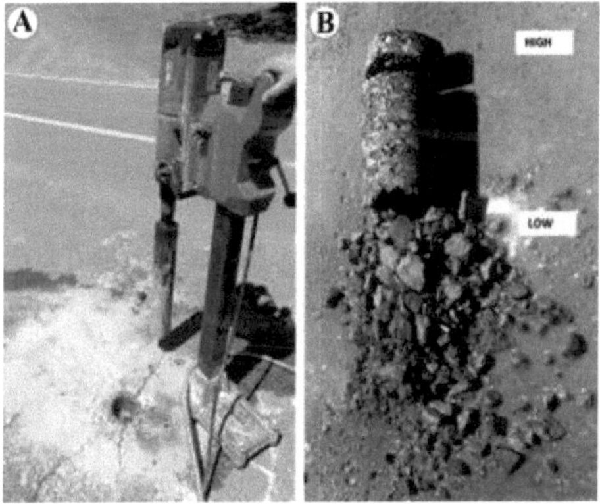

Figure 61(A) Pavement coring operation; (B) Pavement structure sample.

VIII.4.2 Road section N°2 :

The pseudosection presents the results of 2D electrical resistivity measurements carried out on the asphalt pavement showing advanced cracking, characterized by stripping-type damage and cracks in the axis of the road, with erosion of the asphalt pavement at the roadside, as illustrated in the Figure 62

The damage is present along the line, where resistivity values under the defective pavement vary from 400 to 1400 ohms.meter before the winter season, as shown in the Figure 62 (a), and vary from 150 to 700 ohms.meter during the winter season, as shown in Figure 62 (b).

In addition, the results of the pavement coring, revealing the existence of a 4 cm thick layer of bituminous material, highlighted in blue on the figure, resting on a layer of gravelly material, as illustrated in the Figure 63.

Examination of the visual surveys and results mentioned above reveals a number of important points. The surface limestone shows distinct discontinuities, being relatively hard in the middle of the profile but conductive at both ends. In addition, a noticeable decrease in resistivity values was noted for the Figure 62 (a) compared to the Figure 62 (b), occurring both on the surface and at depth during the winter period. This decrease can be attributed to the infiltration of water into the pavement through surface and edge cracks. This infiltration is facilitated by the characteristics of the pavement support soil, which consists of fractured limestone, allowing infiltrated water to circulate. In addition, the current advanced deterioration of the pavement can be attributed to the insufficient thickness of the bituminous layer, which is proving incapable of effectively resisting deterioration.

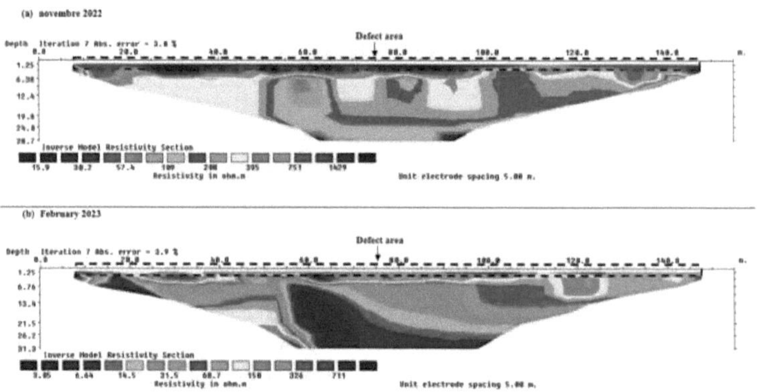

Figure 62(a) 2D resistivity image before the winter season (b) 2D resistivity image during the winter season.

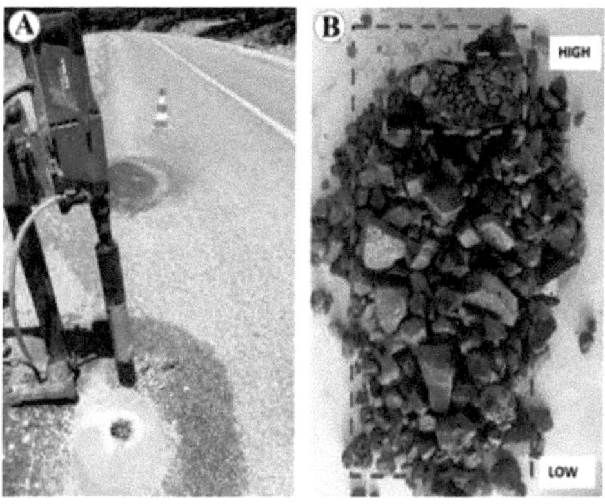

Figure 63(A) Pavement coring operation; (B) Pavement structure sample.

VIII.4.3 Road section N°3 :

The pseudosection illustrates the results of resistivity measurements carried out on an asphalt pavement showing advanced cracks parallel to the road axis, with erosion of the asphalt pavement at the roadside. as illustrated in the Figure 64.

 The damage is present along the line, where resistivity values under the defective pavement vary from 390 to 980 ohms.meter, before the winter season as shown in the profile of the Figure 64 (a) and range from 350 to 880 ohms.m, during the winter season, as shown in the profile in Figure 64 (b).

The results of the pavement coring revealed the existence of a 4 cm thick layer of bituminous material, framed in blue on the figure, resting on gravelly alluvial material. as illustrated in the Figure 65

Examination of the visual inspection and the results obtained reveals a number of important points. Firstly, there is a decrease in surface resistivity values in the Figure 64 (a) compared to the Figure 64 (b) during the winter season. This decrease is attributed to the infiltration of water into the pavement through surface and edge cracks, facilitated by the pavement support soil, consisting of fractured limestone, which allows infiltrated water to circulate. Furthermore, the current state of the asphalt pavement, marked by advanced deterioration, can also be explained by the insufficient thickness of the asphalt layer, which is proving ineffective in resisting deterioration.

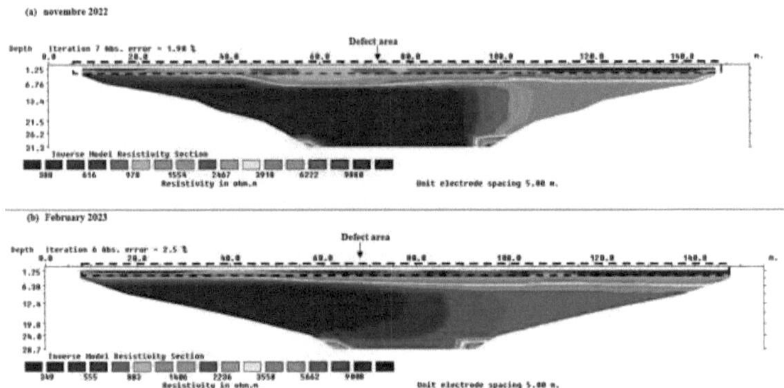

Figure 64(a) 2D resistivity image before the winter season (b) 2D resistivity image during the winter season.

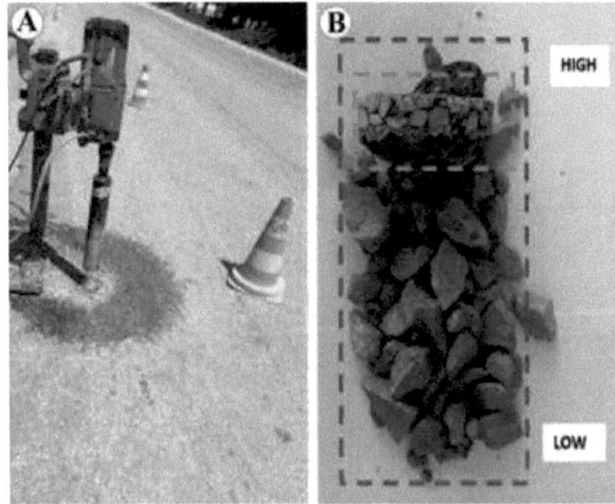

Figure 65(A) Pavement coring operation; (B) Pavement structure sample.

VIII.4.4 Road section N°4 :

The pseudosection shows the results of resistivity measurements carried out on an asphalt pavement showing advanced cracking perpendicular to the road axis, as illustrated in the Figure 66.

 Cracks in the asphalt pavement are present at the beginning of the line over a length of 40 meters, and in the center of the line between 70 meters and 110 meters.

The results of the pavement coring revealed the existence of a 12 cm thick layer of bituminous material, framed in blue on the figure, resting on a sub-layer of gravelly material, as illustrated in the Figure 67.

Analysis of the visual surveys and results detailed above reveals a number of important points. Firstly, the terrain studied exhibits a high degree of homogeneity over a considerable distance, with heterogeneity appearing in particular around 100 metres from the start of the pseudosection, as shown in Figure 66(b), corresponding to the location of a surface water drain. Resistivity values under the defective pavement section range from 21.4 to 22.0 ohms.meter, while the non-defective section shows higher values ranging from 22.0 to 30.8 ohms.meter. In particular, apparent resistivity values drop during the winter season, from 22.0-30.8 ohms.m to 21.4-26.9 ohms.m, attributed to water infiltration through surface and edge cracks. This infiltration leads to an accumulation of moisture on the pavement support soil, mainly composed of clayey silt. The current state of the asphalt pavement, marked by advanced cracking, is attributable to low resistivity values, creating conditions conducive to pavement degradation, particularly near surface water drainage points. In addition, the current thickness of the asphalt layer is insufficient to ensure effective resistance to damage. Conversely, undamaged areas of pavement owe their condition to their location, which minimizes the accumulation of surface water, ensuring rapid drainage of rainwater and reducing the risk of infiltration and pavement degradation.

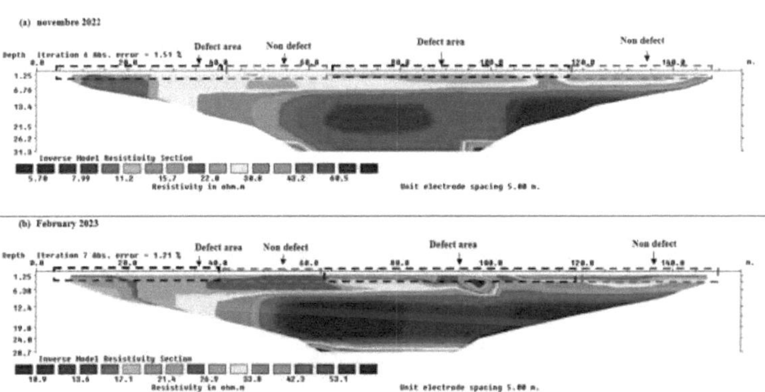

Figure 66(a) 2D resistivity image before the winter season (b) 2D resistivity image during the winter season.

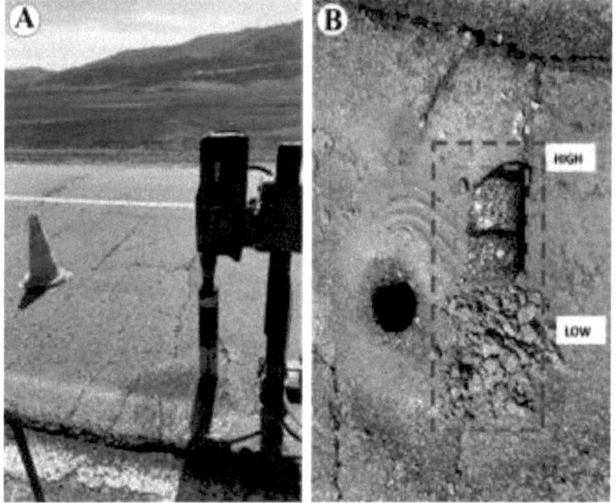

Figure 67(A) Pavement coring operation; (B) Pavement structure sample.

VIII.5 Summary and comparative analysis of electrical resistivity values :

The two tables below summarize the results of the two geophysical campaigns and show that variations in electrical resistivity are associated with different types of pavement failure and seasonal changes.

In particular, examination of the Table 20 allows us to distinguish between areas in poor condition and those in good condition. More specifically, we can observe significant differences between the electrical resistivity values of defective and non-degraded areas in road sections N°1 and N°4. In section N°1, electrical resistivity values in defective areas are considerably lower than those in non-defective areas. This difference can be attributed to the presence of premature cracks, which are not easily detected by visual inspection. In road section 4, on the other hand, the cracks are of an advanced nature, which may explain the relatively low electrical resistivity values in the defective and non defective areas. This finding suggests a more advanced degradation of the road structure in this section.

The results of Table 20 show that 2D ERT can be used conclusively to detect defective areas, which is consistent with previous studies by Orlando et al,[31] Haryati, Alicia[34] and Neyamadpour[35]. Subsequently, in the course of our research, we observed that areas with lower resistivity values are more susceptible to damage.

 The Table 21 on the other hand, highlights the different types of cracks present in four distinct road sections, as well as the variations in electrical resistivity before and during the winter season. One clear observation is the decrease in electrical resistivity values over the winter in all these road sections. In particular, road sections N°1 and N°2 experience significant decreases in electrical resistivity in winter. For road section N°1, this decrease is explained by the presence of premature cracks developing in the bituminous surface of the pavement, underlining the urgency of maintenance work to prevent major deterioration of the road surface under the impact of winter cycles. Similarly, the marked drop in electrical resistivity values in the section of road no. 2 can be explained by the advanced state of cracking of the limestone, which forms the support soil for the pavement, as well as by the advanced deterioration of the bituminous surface of the pavement, favouring the infiltration of rainwater. In view of its advanced state of deterioration, water drainage work and renewal of the pavement structure are required. Road section no. 3 shows a relatively moderate reduction in electrical resistivity values during winter, but resistivity values remain high, indicating that the soil supporting the pavement is resisting winter conditions well. However, the current state of deterioration and cracking of the asphalt mix suggests that the current pavement structure is unsuitable for the traffic on this road. Finally, in the case of road section no. 4, the decrease in electrical resistivity values is relatively small in winter, with generally low values. This is attributable to the advanced state of deterioration, which favours the infiltration of rainwater in winter, increasing the moisture content of the clayey silt support soil. As a result, maintenance work is required, including reinforcement of the supporting soil and renewal of the road surface.

The results in Table 2 reveal a correlation between internal soil moisture, due to seasonal variations, and road infrastructure defects, confirming previous research. In particular, the study by Jackson et al. [36] highlighted this correlation by examining the evolution of the internal soil moisture of a road embankment, monitored using resistivity measurements taken periodically in 2D. These measurements revealed the instability of the road embankment due to seasonal moisture dynamics. In parallel, studies by Chambers et al. [47] and Nobahar et al.[39] also identified a similar relationship by studying the internal moisture dynamics of an embankment, recorded periodically using ERT measurements.

In summary, lower resistivity values are often associated with pavement cracking and the winter season, which may indicate problems related to water infiltration and/or alterations to the pavement structure. These results highlight the potential of electrical resistivity measurements as a tool for assessing pavement condition and monitoring environmental impact, while providing guidance for maintenance and repair decisions.

Table 20Resistivity values for cracked and uncracked zones as a function of pavement failure mode.

	Crack type	Resistivity range (Ω.m)	
		Damaged area	No- Damaged area
Road section N°1	Premature longitudinal and transverse cracking	50 to 95	150 to 300
Road section N°4	Advanced cracking perpendicular to the road axis	21.4 to 22.0	22.0 to 30.8

Table 21Resistivity values before and during winter as a function of pavement failure mode.

	Crack type	Resistivity range (Ω.m)	
		Before winter	during winter
Road section N°1	Premature longitudinal and transverse cracking	150 to 350	50 to 90
Road section N°2	Stripping and advanced cracking along the road axis, with erosion of the roadside pavement.	400 to 1400	150 to 700
Road section N°3	Advanced cracks parallel to the road axis, with erosion of the asphalt pavement at the roadside.	390 to 980	350 to 880
Road section N°4	Advanced cracking perpendicular to the road axis	22.0 to 30.8	21.4 to 26.9

IX. Evaluation of water sensitivity and the impact of thermal cycling on asphalt mixtures with different aggregates and hydrated lime as an additive: Experimental study :

Numerous previous studies have been carried out to assess the water sensitivity and resistance of asphalt mixes to cracking induced by thermal and mechanical stresses, in order to better understand this degradation and select materials with better resistance to fracture and water.

By way of illustration, Li and colleagues [48] studied the low-temperature fracture toughness of 28 bituminous mixtures using the SCB (semi-circular bending test), taking into account various factors such as binder type, modifier, aggregate type, asphalt content and air voids. Test temperature had a significant influence on fracture energy and toughness, showing a shift from brittle to brittle-ductile behavior with increasing temperature. Aggregate type also played a crucial role, with granite-containing mixes having better fracture toughness. Air voids had a negative impact on fracture toughness, and the type of binder modification was also a determining factor.

Another research, conducted by Dehnad and co-authors (2013) [49] investigated the effect of moisture on the permanent deformation of asphalt mixtures under various environmental and traffic conditions, using dynamic creep tests were carried out on saturated and dry asphalt samples with graded dense aggregates. The results showed that, at 40°C with reduced frequency, permanent deformation increased more in saturated samples than in dry samples. Furthermore, at this temperature, humidity has a more negative impact than at 5°C, where the effect of humidity increases with frequency.

Aliha and co-authors (2014) [50] examined how different asphalt characteristics, such as aggregate size and type, bitumen type, and air void content, influence low-temperature mixed fracture toughness (Mode I/II) in various asphalt mixtures, using SCB tests. The results showed that mixes with larger aggregates had better fracture toughness, mainly in mode II (shear). Mixes with calcareous aggregates also showed better toughness than those with siliceous aggregates. Increasing air void content reduced toughness, especially in mixes containing fine siliceous aggregates. In a subsequent study Aliha and co-authors. (2015) [51]investigated the mixed mode I/II low-temperature toughness of five asphalt mixtures modified with various additives, including polyphosphoric acid (PPA), styrene butadiene styrene (SBS), an anti-stripping agent, crumb rubber (CR) and F-T kerosene wax (Sasobit). The results showed that fracture toughness depended on modifier type, air gap percentage and test temperature. In addition, mixed-mode loading proved more critical than pure modes I and II.

Another study [52] evaluated the effect of two additives (liquid anti-stripping agent and hydrated lime) and two modifiers (SBS and PPA) on the moisture sensitivity of asphalt mixtures. Three tests were carried out, including the Lottman AASHTO T283-02 test with five freeze-thaw (FT) cycles, rutting tests and SCB fracture tests. The results of the Lottman test indicated that the liquid anti-stripping agent improved moisture resistance, followed by hydrated lime. The rutting test showed that hydrated lime and SBS modifiers resulted in the lowest rut depth when used in both mixes. The results of the fracture test showed that liquid and hydrated lime produced the highest fracture toughness.

Lamothe and his team [53] carried out a study to assess the damage sustained by hot mix asphalt samples during freeze-thaw cycles under different conditions (dry, partially saturated with water or brine). Samples were subjected to complex modulus tests (E*) after various freeze-thaw cycles to assess the evolution of damage. The results revealed that all samples showed damage, with a much greater severity for those in partially water-saturated conditions. This suggests that increasing salt concentration limits ice formation, thereby reducing the damage caused by freeze-thaw cycles.

Ameri and these **co-workers** [54] investigated the effects of three different additives, namely Evonik, Zycotherm and hydrated lime, on the moisture resistance and other performance characteristics of asphalt mixtures. The results reveal that all three additives improve the moisture resistance of asphalt mixtures, with the mixture containing 0.1% Zycotherm showing the best performance. In addition, hydrated lime at 2% significantly improves the rutting resistance of asphalt mixtures, due to its hardening effect on these mixtures and its hydrophobic property.

Fakhri and colleagues [55] studied the impact of freeze-thaw cycles on the thermal cracking characteristics of saturated asphalt concrete mixtures subjected to mixed mode I/II loading, for which saturated asphalt concrete mixtures were subjected to six freeze-thaw cycles and tested at different temperatures (-5°C, -15°C and -20°C), The results indicate a significant decrease in fracture toughness with increasing freeze-thaw cycles, but stabilization after seven cycles. At lower temperatures, the effective stress intensity factor (KEff) increases, then decreases with further temperature reduction.

Finally, a recent study [56] examines the influence of the amorphous polyalpha-olefin additive (APAO) on the low-temperature (LTC) and intermediate-temperature (ITC) cracking resistance of asphalt mixtures. Tests were carried out under Mode I and II loads, with constant (CT) and variable (VT) temperature cycles. The results show that HMA mixtures containing 6% and 9% APAO exhibit better fracture toughness and higher fracture energy. However, the addition of APAO reduces the flexibility of the blends, but improves their resistance to elastic deformation.

Following on from the above, the aim of our study is to assess the water sensitivity and crack propagation resistance of asphalt mixes. Given the crucial influence of aggregates on the characteristics of bituminous mixtures [57]we have chosen to use two types of aggregate from limestone and shale sources, while incorporating hydrated lime as an additive. These investigations are carried out by means of SCB semicircular bending tests and water sensitivity tests. Asphalt samples are prepared and subjected to water saturation conditions and thermal cycles, with cycle temperatures determined according to the Moroccan climate.

IX.1 Experimental programs :

IX.1.1 Materials :

Two types of aggregate are used in this study. The first mix is made up of aggregates of *limestone* origin, while the second mix is made up of aggregates of *shale* origin. The aggregates used consist of three granular fractions (0/4, 4/6.3 AND 6.3/10). Table 22 presents the aggregate properties for the first mix, while Table 23 shows the properties of the second mix.

The binder used is a pure bitumen with a penetration grade of 35-50, whose properties are summarized in the Table 24.

Table 22 Properties of limestone aggregates :

Tests	Standards	Sand 0/4	Chips 4/6.3	Chippings 6.3/10
Los Angeles (%)	NM EN 1097-2 [58]	-	16	15
Micro-Deval (%)	NM EN 1097-1 [59]	-	8	8
Flattening coefficient (FI %)	NM EN 933-3 [60]	-	5	6
Surface cleanliness (%)	NM 10.1.169 [61]	-	0,8	0,7
Sand equivalent (SE %)	NM EN 933-8 [62]	55	-	-
Fine (% passing 0.08mm)	NM EN 933-1[63]	13.5	-	-
Adhesiveness (%)	NF T66-043-2[64]	-	-	100
MVR density (g/cm3)	NM EN 1097-6 [65]	2,71	2,70	2,70

Table 23 Properties of schist aggregates :

Tests	Standards	Sand 0/4	Chips 4/6.3	Chippings 6.3/10
Los Angeles (%)	NM EN 1097-2 [58]	-	18,0	17,0
Micro-Deval (%)	NM EN 1097-1 [59]	-	22,0	23
Flattening coefficient (FI %)	NM EN 933-3 [60]	-	14,0	12
Surface cleanliness (%)	NM 10.1.169 [61]	-	0,7	0,9
Sand equivalent (SE %)	NM EN 933-8 [62]	45	-	-
Fine (% passing 0.08mm)	NM EN 933-1[63]	13.02	-	-
Adhesiveness (%)	NF T66-043-2[64]	-	-	100
MVR density (g/cm3)	NM EN 1097-6 [65]	2,61	2,63	2,64

Table 24 Bitumen properties :

Tests	Standards	Results
Needle penetration (10th mm)	NM EN 1426 [3]	44.0
Determination of softening point (°C)	NM EN 1427 [4]	58.0
Relative density (g/cm3)	NM EN 15326 [66]	1,04
Flash point (°C)	NM EN ISO 2592 [18]	307
Open vessel fire point (°C)	NM EN ISO 2592 [18]	312

IX.1.2 Mix design :

In order to determine the optimum composition of asphalt mix for a wearing course with a nominal maximum aggregate size of 10 mm, asphalt mix design tests were carried out in accordance with the recommendations of the Moroccan guideline for hot mix asphalt materials [5]. The Figure 68 shows the granular curves of the two mixes, while Table 25 shows the characteristics of the asphalt mixes tested. The optimum bitumen dosages for mix N°1 and mix N°2 were identified as 5.7% and 5.9% respectively.

In addition, a 2% hydrated lime additive was incorporated into both aggregate mixes as a filler, whether from limestone or shale sources. Minor adjustments to aggregate proportions were made to maintain the same actual mass volumes as those of mixes N°1 and N°2. The binder was then introduced to prepare mixes N°3 and N°4, following the same optimum bitumen dosages.

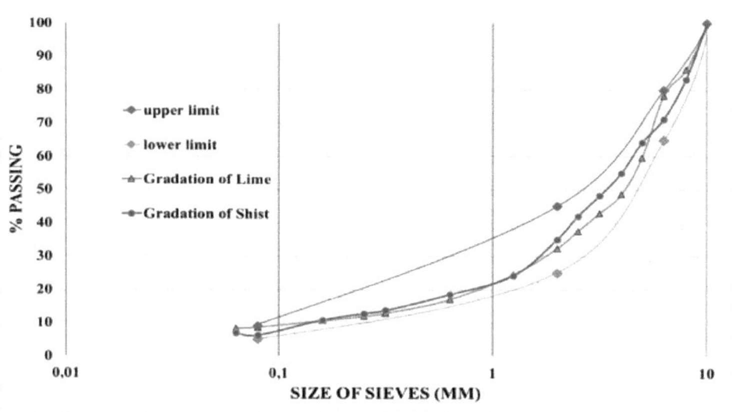

Figure 68shows the granular curves of granular mixtures.

Table 25:shows the aggregate and bitumen proportions of the asphalt mixes tested.

	Limestone mix N°1	Schist Mix N° 2	Lime & limestone mix N°3	Schist & Lime Mix N°4
Sand 0/4	50,00%	48,00%	49,00%	47,00%
Chips 4/6.3	24,00%	25,00%	23,50%	24,50%
Chippings 6.3/10	26,00%	27,00%	25,50%	26,50%
Additive (hydrated lime)	-	-	2%	2%
bitumen (%)	5,7	5,9	5,7	5,9
MVR [67]	2,49	2,42	2,49	2,42

IX.1.3 Water resistance test:

Water resistance tests were carried out in accordance with NM EN 12697-12 [17]method B, to assess the water sensitivity of bituminous mixes. At least ten samples were required for each type of mix. The samples were manufactured by applying a load of 60 kN for 300 ± 5 seconds, and the percentage of air voids in the prepared samples is around 6%.

The samples were divided into two equivalent batches. The first batch, containing the "dry samples", was stored at a temperature of 18°C ± 1 and a humidity of 50% ± 10 for a period of 7 days. The second batch of "wet test tubes" is subjected to a degassing process with water saturation, as follows: For approximately 1 hour ± 5 minutes, the specimens were exposed to a residual pressure of 47 kPa ± 5% using a vacuum pump. Water was then introduced until the specimens were completely immersed, while maintaining the residual pressure of 47 kPa ± 5%. The specimens were kept immersed for 2 hours at the same pressure, then stored in water at a temperature of 18°C ± 1 for 7 days.

The wet and dry test specimens were then subjected to compression testing with a monotonic displacement-controlled load of 50 mm/min. Simple compressive strength was determined from the maximum load at failure of the test specimen, expressed in megapascals, and represented by the average of five measurements.

The water resistance of the specimens, noted i/C, is described by the ratio of the average resistance of the wet batch (Cw) to the average resistance of the dry batch (Cd) according toEquation 19 as follows

Equation 19Water resistance :

$$\frac{i}{C} = 100 \times \frac{Cw}{Cd}$$

To meet water resistance criteria, a minimum value of 75% is recommended.

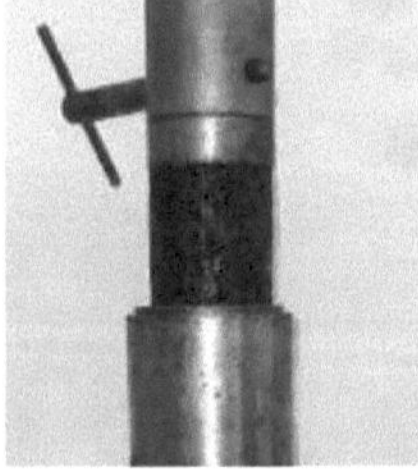

Figure 69:Compression test on a single specimen

IX.1.4 SCB test: Semi-Circular Bending test:

The SCB (Semi-Circular Bending test) is based on the principle of three-point bending applied to half-cylinder samples, each with a central crack [28]. The geometry of the SCB semi-circular bending test specimens for Mode I, characterized by thickness (t), radius (r), crack length (a) and distance between the two steel supports (2S), was adjusted to 0.8 times the diameter of the specimen (0.8d) subjected to load (P), as illustrated below.

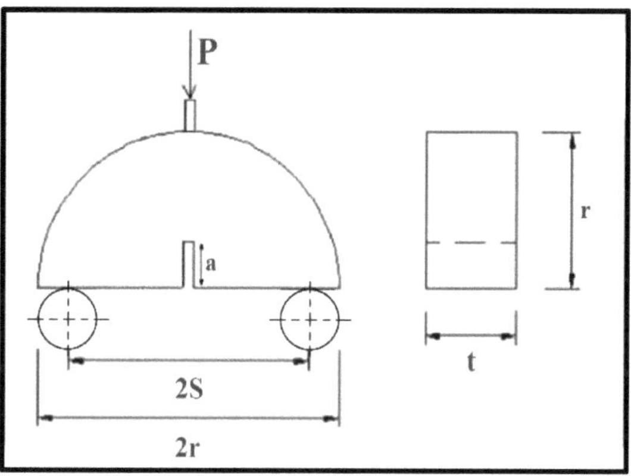

Figure 70Geometry of SCB semicircular bending samples for mode I.

To prepare these samples, we use a PCG gyratory shear press, conforming to standard NF EN 12697-31. This method enables us to control various parameters such as air void percentage, density, specimen height and other mechanical characteristics of bituminous mixes, thus guaranteeing uniform mechanical properties.

For this purpose, asphalt samples are prepared and compacted to obtain asphalt specimens with a final void percentage of 5%. The preparation method consists of placing laboratory-prepared asphalt mixes at test temperature (approx. 160°C) in a 150 mm cylindrical mold. A vertical pressure of 0.6 MPa, inclined at a slight angle of around 1°, is applied to the top of the specimen, while imparting a circular movement. These combined actions result in compaction by kneading. Density (and void percentage reduction) improves progressively with the number of rotations.

Once the asphalt samples have been obtained, we cut them into slices averaging 50 mm in thickness, using a high-speed rotary cutter equipped with a blade. Each slice is then divided into two equal semicircular samples, with an average height of 72 mm. For the SCB test, we then apply vertical cracks to the center of the semicircular samples. These cracks are (3.0 ± 1.0) mm wide and (10.0 ± 1.0) mm deep.   The steps involved in manufacturing the SCB test specimens are illustrated in the following figure:

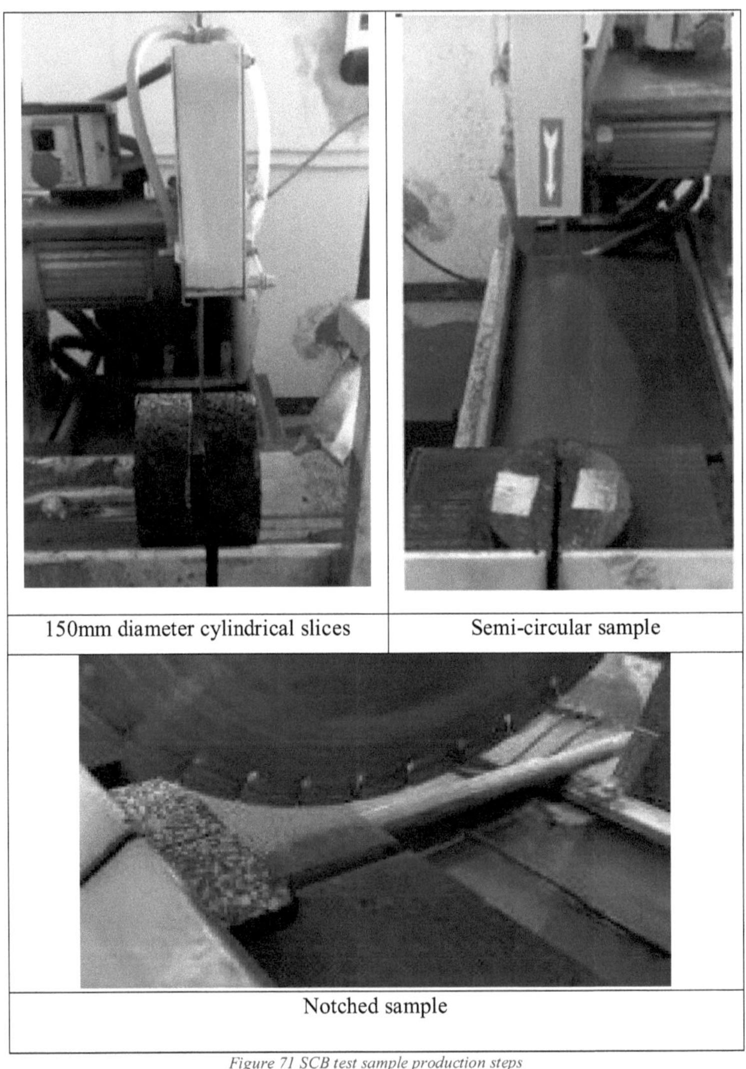

Figure 71 SCB test sample production steps

The samples are then subjected to a degassing treatment with water saturation using the following procedure: For approximately 1 hour ± 5 minutes, the specimens were exposed to a residual pressure of 47 kPa ± 5% using a vacuum pump. Water was then introduced until the specimens were completely immersed, while maintaining a residual pressure of 47 kPa ± 5%. The specimens were kept immersed for 2 hours at the same pressure, and then stored in plastic sample bags to preserve their water content.

During the test, deformation evolved at a constant loading rate of 1.27mm/min. However, it is important to note that the fracture energy showed consistent behavior over a range of loading rates from 1mm/min to 5mm/min, and the tests demonstrated high repeatability with a low coefficient of variation (COV) [68].

Simultaneously, the associated load increases until it reaches a maximum value (Pmax), and the load-displacement curve reveals four main segments: the stiffness zone, the strength zone, the toughness zone and the softening zone, as shown in Figure. 72. The cumulative work performed in these zones contributes to the fracture energy [69,70] . It is essential to point out that this study does not focus on the calculation of fracture energy; rather, it evaluates the fracture resistance of asphalt mixes for SCB geometry using fracture toughness (K_{Ic}) as the main parameter of the fracture test.

Fracture toughness represents the highest maximum value of the stress intensity factor when cracking occurs [71] . The application of the stress intensity factor (SIF) to asphalt concrete stems from the pioneering work of Lim et al. (1993)[72]. Subsequent research by Abu et al. (2014)[36] explored and validated its relevance to heterogeneous asphalt materials. The stress intensity factor is now incorporated into current standards for SCB testing, as shown in EN 12697-44:2019[73].

Mode I fracture toughness (K_{Ic}) was calculated on the basis of the work of Lim et al. (1993)[35] and standards EN 12697-44: 2019[73]:

$$\sigma_{\mathbf{max}} = \frac{P_{\mathrm{max}}}{2r\times t} \; \mathrm{N/mm^2} \qquad\qquad \textit{Equation 20Maximum stress}$$

$$K_{Ic} = \sigma_{max}.Y_1.\sqrt{\pi a}\; \;^{N}\!/_{mm^{3}/_2} \qquad\qquad \textit{Equation 21fracture toughness}$$

$$Y_1 = 4.782 - 1.219\left(\frac{a}{r}\right) + 0.063\exp\left(7.045\left(\frac{a}{r}\right)\right) \qquad \textit{Equation 22normalized stress intensity factor}$$

Where

- ✓ $\sigma_{\mathbf{max}}$ is the maximum stress applied ;
- ✓ $P_{\mathbf{max}}$ is the maximum load applied ;
- ✓ Y_1 is the normalized stress intensity factor, calculated using equation (4) for the ratio between span and radius, s/r = 0.8; and all parameters are described in the previous paragraphs.

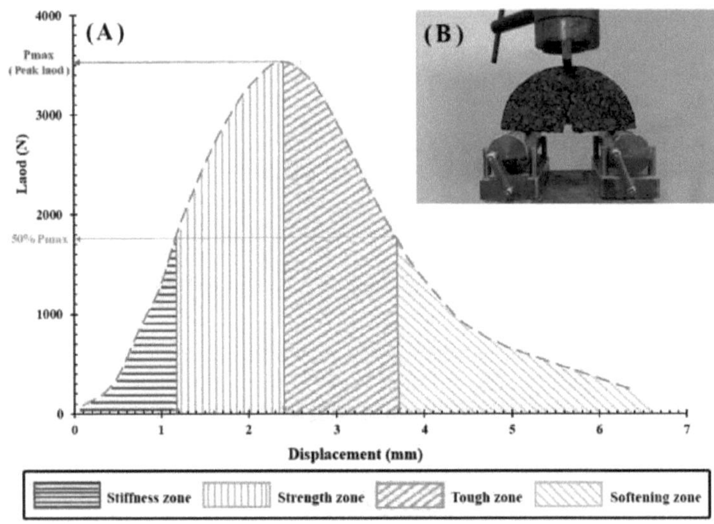

Figure. 72. A) Representative load-displacement curve obtained for one of the asphalt mixes tested, together with other fracture indices B) Experimental set-up used to test semicircular specimens under three-point bending load.

IX.1.5 Thermal cycles

In order to ensure consistency and similarity between field and test conditions, while enabling a thorough assessment of the impact of water saturation and temperature variations on the resistance of asphalt mixes to cracking, we chose to select temperature values commonly observed on Moroccan pavements.

According to the study by Lagrini et al (2020) [11]average temperatures in Morocco generally range from -5°C to +20°C, with peaks of +40°C. These extreme temperatures were considered to be the most restrictive and were used to define thermal cycle temperatures.

To this end, the prepared samples were placed inside a climatic chamber, where they were subjected to temperature variations. Each cycle had a total duration of 13 hours, comprising 6 hours of constant temperature maintenance for each stage, plus one hour of temperature variation at a rate of 50°C/h (30 minutes of cooling and 30 minutes of heating). The Figure 73 illustrates temperature control within the thermal chamber and Figure 74 shows the climatic chamber used to apply the thermal cycles. The characteristics of this climatic chamber allow automatic programming of thermal cycles, and the reference of this climatic chamber is 10-D1429/A(controls), with a temperature range of -25 to 70°C.

114

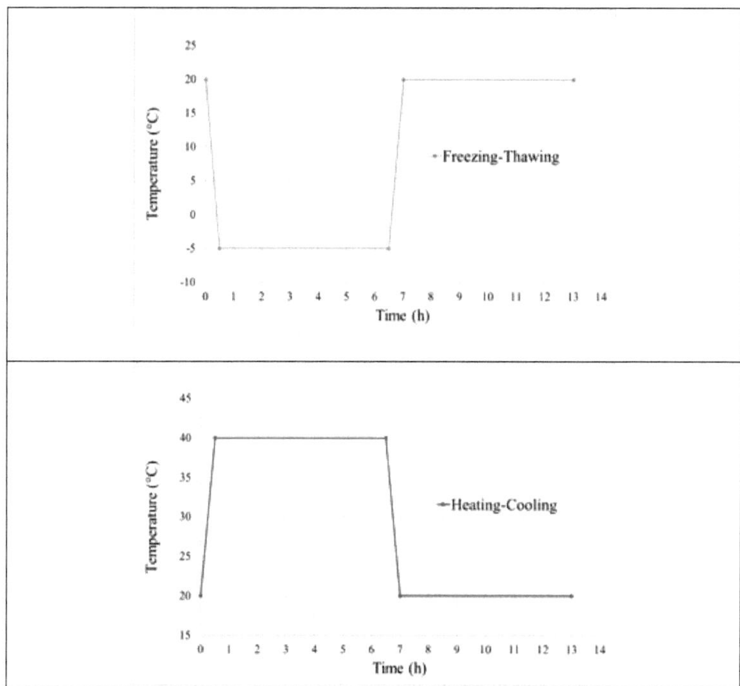

Figure 73 Thermal enclosure control temperature for FT AND HC cycle.

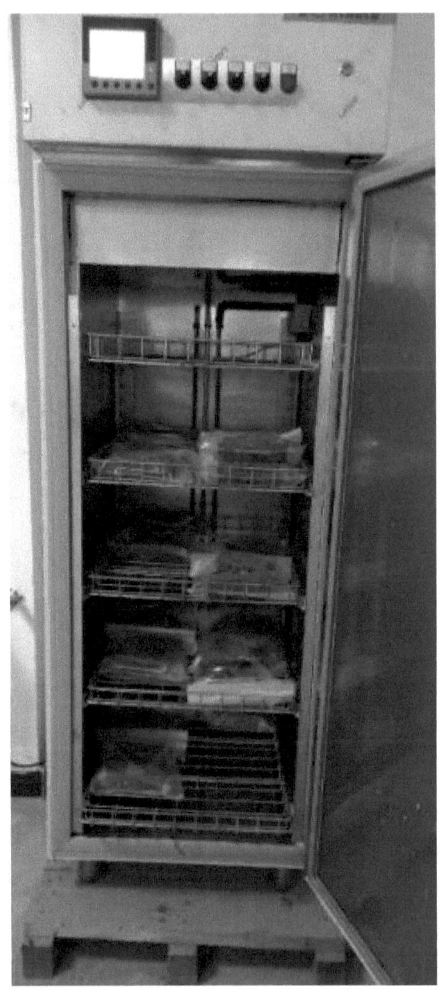

Figure 74climatic chamber

Subsequently, three conditioning methods were chosen, as shown in Figures 75, 76 and 77. The first method involves the use of Freeze-Thaw cycles with a temperature variation from 20°C (for 6 hours) to -5°C (for 6 hours). The second method involves the use of Heating-Cooling cycles with temperature variations from 20°C (for 6 hours) to 40°C (for 6 hours). Finally, the third method consists of using freeze-thaw cycles followed by heating-cooling cycles (Freeze-Thaw then Heating-Cooling), where samples were subjected to 60 thermal cycles ranging from -5°C (for 6 hours) to 20°C (for 6 hours) continuously, followed by a temperature variation from 20°C (for 6 hours) to 40°C (for 6 hours).

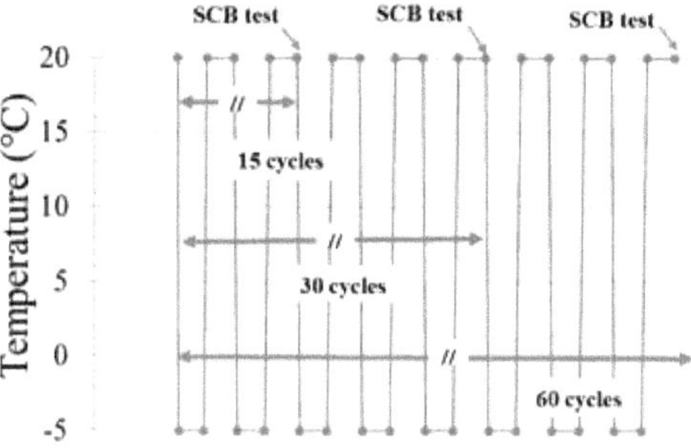

Figure 75FT thermal cycling profiles imposed on samples subjected to the SCB test

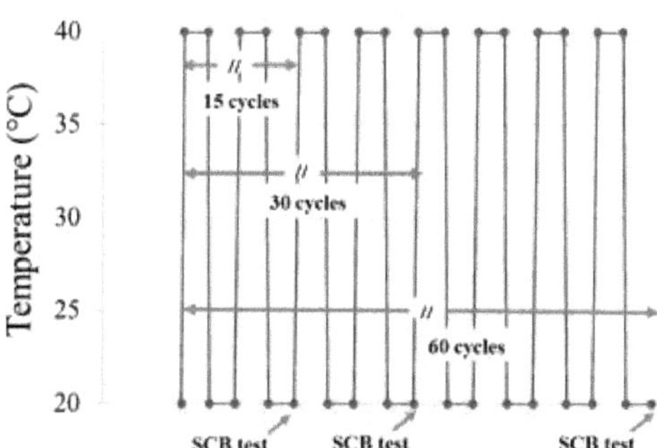

Figure 76FT-HT thermal cycling profiles for SCB test specimens

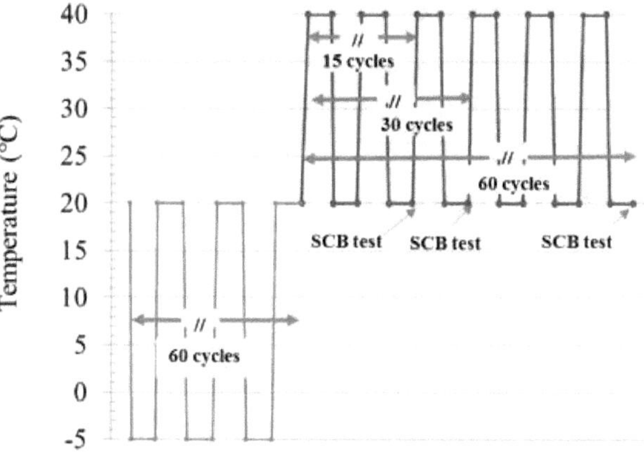

Figure 77FT-HT thermal cycling profiles for SCB test specimens

The SCB samples were then tested after 15, 30 and 60 cycles respectively for the FT (Freeze-Thaw) and HT (Heating-Cooling) thermal cycles, and after 75, 90 and 120 cycles for the FT-HT (Freeze-Thaw then Heating-Cooling) thermal cycle. A total of 160 SCB samples were tested. At the end of each cycle sequence, four SCB samples were fractured at a temperature of 20°C. Toughness was calculated by taking the average of the four recorded values. It is essential to note that a series of samples were tested in their initial state, without having been subjected to thermal cycling. The Figure 78 shows the flow chart of the experimental program implemented as part of this study.

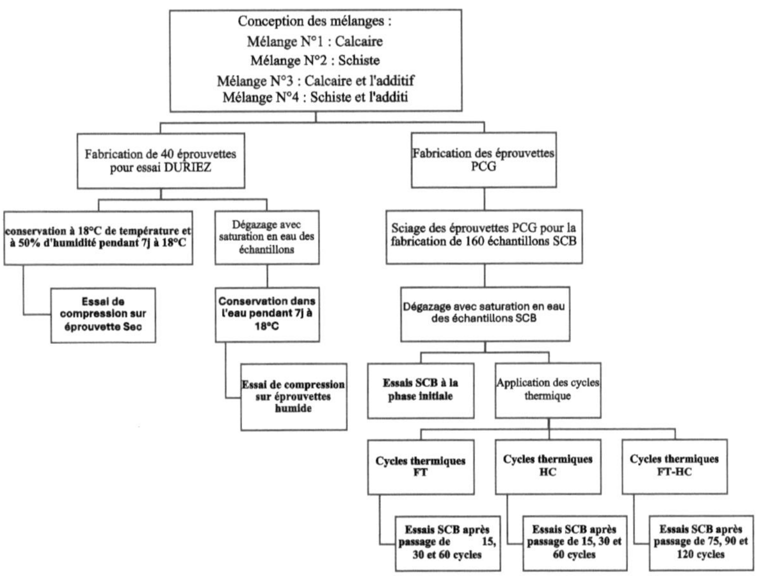

Figure 78Flow chart of the experimental program for this study.

IX.2 Test results for water sensitivity and fracture toughness:

IX.2.1 Water sensitivity test for bituminous mixes :

The Figure 79 shows the results of the compressive strength of hot mix asphalt mixes made from shale or limestone aggregates, as well as those containing hydrated lime as an additive, evolving as a function of dry or wet storage conditions.

As expected, the strength of the samples under dry conditions is higher than the strength of the wet samples for each material. Furthermore, the addition of hydrated lime increases sample strength in both cases, for both shale and limestone. This improvement in strength is most notable for shale, where compressive strength increases significantly in the presence of hydrated lime.

Comparatively speaking, limestone has a higher initial strength than shale, and retains this superiority even after the addition of hydrated lime. However, the addition of hydrated lime also improves the strength of limestone.

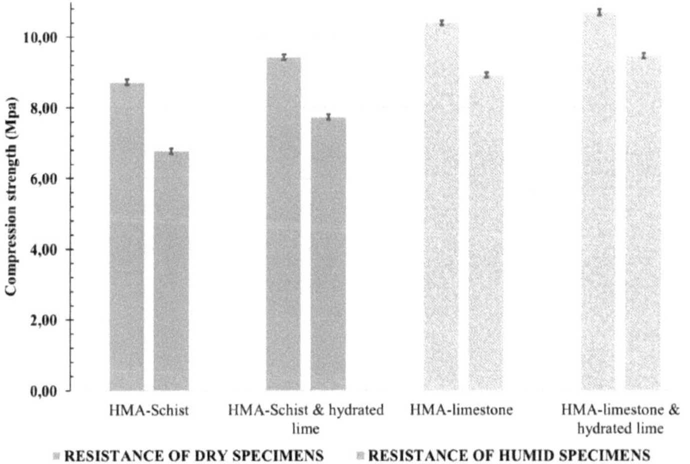

Figure 79Compressive strength in dry and wet conditions.

The Figure 80 shows the results of the evaluation of the water resistance of asphalt mixtures described by the ratio (i/C) as a function of the nature of the shale or limestone aggregates, as well as those containing hydrated lime as an additive.

Although all samples have (i/C) values above 75%. However, resistance to water-induced damage increases for each sample with the addition of hydrated lime.

Limestone and limestone & hydrated lime initially have higher strength ratios than shale and shale & hydrated lime. However, even though the strength ratio of shale is initially lower, the addition of hydrated lime has a greater impact on improving strength, resulting in an increase in the ratio. The strong adhesion between bitumen and aggregates in the case of mixes modified with hydrated lime is the reason for better performance [54,74].

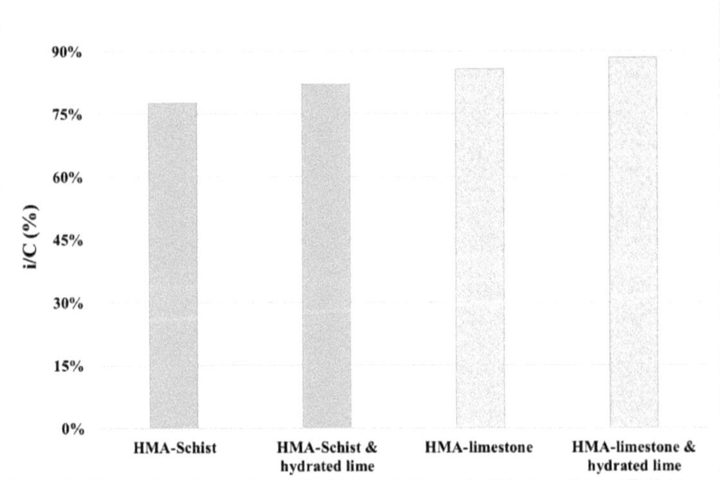

Figure 80(i/C) ratio values for various asphalt mix samples

IX.2.2 Impact of Thermal Cycling on Fracture Toughness :

The Figure 81 shows how the average fracture toughness of asphalt mixes made from shale and limestone aggregates, as well as those containing hydrated lime as an additive, evolves as a function of the number of thermal cycles (FT) applied, ranging from -5 to 20°C. Fracture toughness decreases as the number of cycles increases, whatever the type of aggregate.

For asphalt produced from shale, fracture toughness decreases by 20.7% compared with the initial value after 60 cycles. When hydrated lime is added to asphalt mixes made from shale aggregates, fracture toughness decreases by 14.9% after 60 cycles. Figure 81 (a).

For asphalt produced from limestone, strength decreases by 13.3% after 60 cycles, while the addition of lime to asphalt produced from limestone aggregates results in a decrease of 11.8% after 60 cycles. Figure 81 (b).

In addition, asphalt mixes with the additive (hydrated lime) have a higher strength than those without. This increase in strength varies from 13.7% to 19.6% for asphalt made from shale aggregates and from 4.5% to 6.2% for asphalt made from limestone aggregates, depending on the number of thermal cycles.

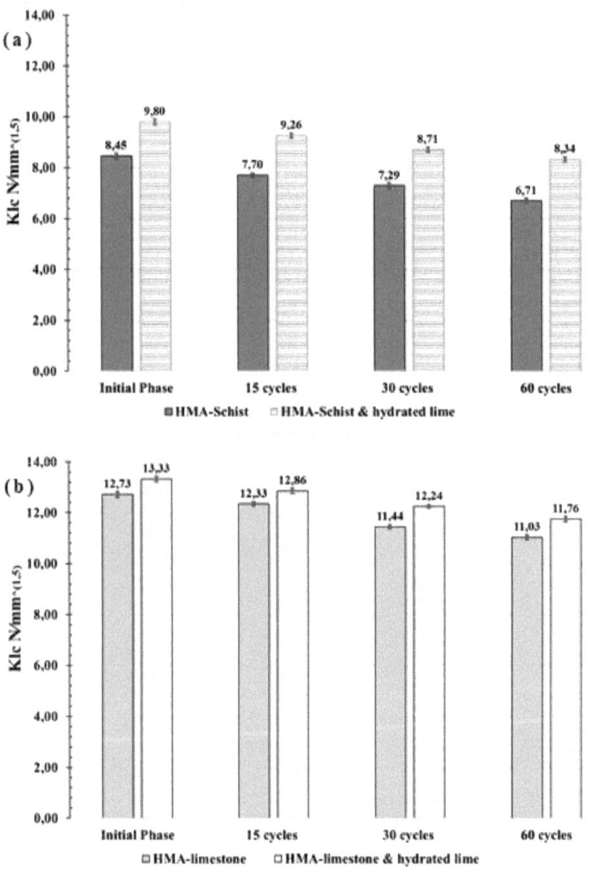

Figure 81 Fracture toughness values of asphalt mix after application of a thermal cycle FT a) Asphalt made from shale b) Asphalt made from limestone.

IX.2.3 Impact of Thermal Cycles (H.C.) on Fracture Toughness :

The Figure 82 shows how the strength of asphalt mixes made from shale and limestone aggregates, as well as those containing hydrated lime as an additive, changes as a function of the number of thermal cycles (HT) applied, ranging from 20 to 40°C. Fracture toughness decreases as the number of cycles increases, whatever the type of aggregate.

For asphalt produced from shale, fracture toughness decreases by 25.6% compared with the initial value after 60 cycles. When hydrated lime is added to asphalt mixes made from shale aggregates, fracture toughness decreases by 20.2% after 60 cycles. Figure 82(a).

For asphalt produced from limestone, strength decreases by 13.6% after 60 cycles, while the addition of lime to asphalt produced from limestone aggregates results in a 13% decrease after 60 cycles. Figure 82 (b).

In addition, asphalt mixes with the additive (hydrated lime) have a higher strength than those without. This increase in strength varies from 13.7% to 19.5% for asphalt made from shale aggregates and from 4.5% to 5.2% for asphalt made from limestone aggregates, depending on the number of thermal cycles.

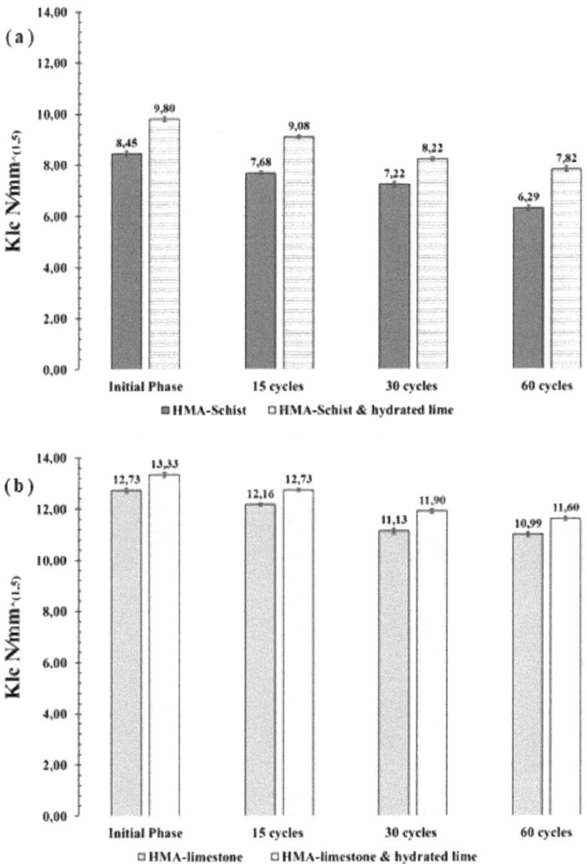

Figure 82Asphalt fracture toughness values after HC thermal cycling
a)   Asphalt made from shale b) Asphalt made from limestone.

IX.2.4 Impact of Thermal Cycles (F.T.-H.C.) on Fracture Toughness :

The Figure 83 shows how the strength of asphalt mixes made from shale and limestone aggregates, as well as those containing hydrated lime as an additive, evolves as a function of the number of thermal cycles (FT-HT) applied, ranging from 20 to 40°C after 60 continuous cycles from -5 to 20°C as defined above. It can be seen that fracture toughness decreases as the number of cycles increases, whatever the type of aggregate.

For asphalt produced from shale, fracture toughness decreases by 37% compared with the initial value after 120 cycles. When hydrated lime is added to asphalt mixes made from shale aggregates, fracture toughness decreases by 29% after 120 cycles.

For asphalt produced from limestone, strength decreases by 24.5% after 120 cycles, while the addition of lime to asphalt produced from limestone aggregates results in a 21.3% decrease after 120 cycles.

In addition, asphalt mixes with the additive (hydrated lime) have a higher strength than those without. This increase in strength varies from 15.9% to 30.6% for asphalt mixes made from shale aggregates and from 4.7% to 9.2% for asphalt mixes made from limestone aggregates, depending on the number of thermal cycles.

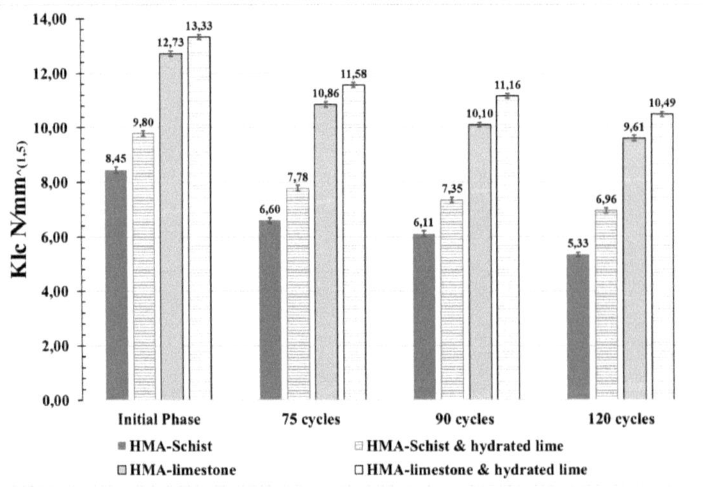

Figure 83Asphalt fracture toughness values after HC thermal cycling

IX.3 Summary Comparative analysis of fracture toughness for various thermal cycles:

When examining fracture toughness data for different thermal cycle conditions (FT, HT, FT-HT), it is clear that asphalt strength decreases as the number of thermal cycles increases. This trend suggests a reduction in the ability of asphalt mixes to withstand repeated thermal variations.

Freeze-thaw cycles impose increased stress on samples, leading to a reduction in their fracture resistance. In addition, during the thaw phase, water particles migrate to the interface between the binder and the aggregates, weakening the cohesion of this interface [55]. further research has highlighted the formation of microcracks in the binder due to the tendency of the asphalt matrix to contract more than the aggregates [55,75,76]This differential contraction between the asphalt matrix and the aggregates contributes to reducing the asphalt's breaking strength.

The impact of heating-cooling (HC) cycles results in reduced adhesion between aggregate and binder, which increases the susceptibility of asphalt mixes to deformation, thus explaining the reduction in breaking strength.

In addition, high temperature cycles (HT from 20 to 40°C) have a more adverse effect on asphalt strength than low temperature cycles (FT from -5 to 20°C). This difference is due to the viscoelastic properties of the binder and the interface between binder and aggregate, which react significantly to temperature variations. At higher temperatures, the binder adopts a viscous behavior, while at lower temperatures it becomes predominantly elastic (or brittle). This results in greater resistance to fracture and, consequently, more energy is required to break the binder. [51,55,77]   .

When FT and HT cycles are combined (FT-HT), asphalt mixes suffer increased damage, resulting from the formation of microcracks in the binder after FT cycles, and loss of adhesion between binder and aggregate during HT cycles.

For example, for asphalt mixes made from shale, the reduction in fracture toughness is generally more pronounced than for those made from limestone. This means that shale-based hot mix asphalt is less resistant to thermal cycling.

However, asphalt mixes containing lime as an additive generally show higher strength than those without. For shale-based mixes, this improvement is generally between 13.3% and 30.6%, while for limestone-based mixes, it varies from 4.5% to 9.2%. It should be noted that this increase in strength is more pronounced for shale-based asphalt than for limestone-based asphalt.

The incorporation of hydrated lime as an additive in asphalt results in several significant performance improvements. Firstly, it promotes the precipitation of calcium ions on the surface of aggregates, which enhances the adhesion of asphalt to bitumen[78].

In addition, hydrated lime reduces asphalt's tendency to deform at high temperatures, particularly in its early stages of use, when it is most susceptible to rutting damage. This improvement results from the reinforcement of the asphalt film through the incorporation of hydrated lime. Lime also strengthens the bond between asphalt and aggregates in hot-mix asphalt (HMA), making it less susceptible to the damaging effects of moisture. This collaboration has a considerable effect on increasing the resistance of hot-mix asphalt to rutting. As asphalt ages due to oxidation, hydrated lime has a dual beneficial effect. On the one hand, it slows down the oxidation process, and on the other, it mitigates the damage caused by oxidation by-products. As a result, asphalt retains its flexibility, preventing it from becoming excessively vulnerable to cracking, whether due to fatigue or low-temperature conditions. The filling effect of hydrated lime dispersed in asphalt acts synergistically to improve fracture resistance and further strengthen asphalt's resistance to cracking [74].

X.   Conclusion and recommendation:

In conclusion, this study highlighted the usefulness of electrical resistivity tomography (ERT) in assessing the condition of bituminous pavements in Morocco. We established a direct correlation between the electrical resistivity of the soil and the cracking of the asphalt wearing course, taking into account the measurement periods before and during the winter season. By combining ERT with visual inspection and coring, we have increased our understanding of the factors contributing to pavement degradation, facilitating targeted maintenance and repair intervention.

Electrical resistivity tomography campaigns carried out at different times on road sections offer non-destructive assessment and monitoring, enabling early detection of vulnerable areas and promoting proactive maintenance. This translates into reduced costs and improved pavement durability, contributing to user safety.

It's important to note that while ERT is a useful tool, it needs to be complemented by other geophysical survey methods, such as ground penetrating radar (GPR), for a complete assessment of pavement component interfaces.

With regard to the study on the impact of thermal cycling and the addition of hydrated lime on asphalt mixtures, several important conclusions were drawn. Firstly, all samples met water resistance specifications, but the addition of hydrated lime increased resistance to water damage, particularly for shale-based samples. In addition, thermal cycles clearly demonstrated their influence on the fracture toughness of asphalt mixes, underlining the importance of taking these constraints into account in pavement design and maintenance, especially in a climate as varied as that of Morocco. Finally, the results indicate that shale-based asphalt mixes are more vulnerable to thermal cycling than limestone-based mixes, but the addition of hydrated lime was beneficial for both types of asphalt.

However, we would point out the importance of exploring other innovative materials and additives that could further improve the durability and damage resistance of asphalt mixes, taking into account specific local climatic conditions.

In summary, this study highlights the importance of material selection, the addition of additives such as hydrated lime, and the consideration of local climatic conditions in the design and construction of durable pavements. These results provide valuable information for engineers and road construction professionals to improve the strength and durability of pavements in different climatic conditions.

References :

[1] Mehdi MA, Cherradi T, Bouyahyaoui A, El Karkouri S, Qachar A. Evolution of a flexible pavement deterioration, analyzing the road inspections results. Materials Today: Proceedings 2022;58:1222-8. https://doi.org/10.1016/j.matpr.2022.01.452.

[2] Barillot J, Cabanes H, Carillo P. Roads and their pavements manual public works 2018.

[3] NM EN 1426. Bitumen and bituminous binders - Determination of needle penetration 2019.

[4] NM EN 1427. Bitumen and bituminous binders - Determination of the softening point - Ring and Ball method 2019.

[5] Moroccan Ministry of Public Works. Directive for hot mix asphalt materials n.d.

[6] NF P 98-086. Structural design of road pavements Application to new pavements 2011.

[7] H. Di Benedetto, J.-F. Corté. Bituminous road materials 2: composition and thermomechanical properties of mixtures. Lavoisier 2004.

[8] Directorate General of Metrology. Morocco Climate Report 2023.

[9] Rhanem M. The esparto grass (Stipa tenacissima L.) in the Midelt plain (upper Moulouya watershed, Morocco) - Elements of climatology. physio-geo 2009:1-20. https://doi.org/10.4000/physio-geo.696.

[10] Directorate General of Metrology. Morocco Climate Report 2007.

[11] Lagrini K, Ghafiri A, Ouali A, Elrhaz K, Feddoul R, Elmoutaki S. Application of geographical information system (GIS) for the development of climatological air temperature vulnerability maps: An example from Morocco. Meteorological Applications 2020;27. https://doi.org/10.1002/met.1871.

[12] Ionesco T, Mathez J, Rouge JF, ill. Climatology, bioclimatology and phytogeography of Morocco 1966.

[13] NF P 98-086. Structural design of road pavements Application to new pavements 2019.

[14] Sarroukh M, Lahlou K, Farah M, Mequedade N, Mamoune MBE. Calculation of equivalent temperature according to Moroccan climate and its effect on pavement design 2020;38.

[15] LCPC 2007. Manual LPC d'aide à la formulation des enrobés 2007.

[16] EN 12697-31. Bituminous mixtures - Test methods - Part 31: specimen preparation by gyratory compactor 2018.

[17] NM EN 12697-12. Bituminous mixtures - Test methods - Part 12: determination of the water sensitivity of bituminous specimens 2018.

[18] NM ISO 2592. Petroleum and related products - Determination of flash and fire points - Cleveland open cup method 2017.

[19] CEREMA. Diagnosis and design of pavement reinforcements,. 2016.

[20] manual for the reinforcement of coated pavements n.d.

[21] FISSAA Smail. Use of GPR (Ground Penetrating Radar) in road applications n.d.

[22] Samouëlian A, Cousin I, Tabbagh A, Bruand A, Richard G. Electrical resistivity survey in soil science: a review. Soil and Tillage Research 2005;83:173-93. https://doi.org/10.1016/j.still.2004.10.004.

[23] LCPC. Le catalog des dégradations de surface des chaussées. 1998.

[24] KHAWAJA H, AHMAD T. Review of Low-Temperature Crack (LTC) Developments in Asphalt Pavements. IJM 2018;12. https://doi.org/10.21152/1750-9548.12.2.169.

[25] Les pathologies de voirie. tp.demain n.d. https://tpdemain.com/module/les-pathologies-de-voirie/ (accessed March 14, 2024).

[26] Wagoner M, Buttlar W, Paulino G. Development of a Single-Edge Notched Beam Test for Asphalt Concrete Mixtures. Journal of Testing and Evaluation 2005;33:452-60. https://doi.org/10.1520/JTE12579.

[27] Al-Qadi IL, Scarpas T, Loizos A. Pavement Cracking: Mechanisms, Modeling, Detection, Testing and Case Histories. CRC Press; 2008.

[28] Lu DX, Bui HH, Saleh M. Effects of specimen size and loading conditions on the fracture behaviour of asphalt concretes in the SCB test. Engineering Fracture Mechanics 2021;242:107452. https://doi.org/10.1016/j.engfracmech.2020.107452.

[29] Badeli S, Carter A, Doré G. Effect of laboratory compaction on the viscoelastic characteristics of an asphalt mix before and after rapid freeze-thaw cycles. Cold Regions Science and Technology 2018;146:98-109. https://doi.org/10.1016/j.coldregions.2017.12.001.

[30] Caro S, Masad E, Bhasin A, Little DN. Moisture susceptibility of asphalt mixtures, Part 1: mechanisms. International Journal of Pavement Engineering 2008;9:81-98. https://doi.org/10.1080/10298430701792128.

[31] Orlando L, Cardarelli E, Cercato M, De Donno G, Di Giambattista L. Pavement testing by integrated geophysical methods: Feasibility, resolution and diagnostic potential. Journal of Applied Geophysics 2017;136:462-73. https://doi.org/10.1016/j.jappgeo.2016.11.024.

[32] Alsharahi G, Filali Bouami M, Faize A, Louzazni M, Khamlichi A, Atounti M. Contribution of analysis and detection the risks appearing in roads using GPR method: A case study in Morocco. Ain Shams Engineering Journal 2021;12:1435-50. https://doi.org/10.1016/j.asej.2020.10.014.

[33] Chambers et al. - 2014 - 4D electrical resistivity tomography monitoring of.pdf n.d.

[34] Haryati A, Alicia D. Geophysical Characterisation of Road Subsurface. InCIEC 2014 2014. https://doi.org/10.1007/978-981-287-290-6_41.

[35] Neyamadpour A. Detection of subsurface cracking depth using electrical resistivity tomography: A case study in Masjed-Soleiman, Iran. Construction and Building Materials 2018;191:1103-8. https://doi.org/10.1016/j.conbuildmat.2018.10.027.

[36] Jackson PD, Northmore KJ, Meldrum PI, Gunn DA, Hallam JR, Wambura J, et al. Non-invasive moisture monitoring within an earth embankment - a precursor to failure. NDT & E International 2002;35:107-15. https://doi.org/10.1016/S0963-8695(01)00030-5.

[37] Rasul H, Zou L, Olofsson B. Monitoring of moisture and salinity content in an operational road structure by electrical resistivity tomography: Monitoring of moisture and salinity content. Near Surface Geophysics 2018;16:423-44. https://doi.org/10.1002/nsg.12002.

[38] Diallo MC, Cheng LZ, Rosa E, Gunther C, Chouteau M. Integrated GPR and ERT data interpretation for bedrock identification at Cléricy, Québec, Canada. Engineering Geology 2019;248:230-41. https://doi.org/10.1016/j.enggeo.2018.09.011.

[39] Nobahar M, Salunke R, Alzeghoul OE, Khan MS, Amini F. Mapping of Slope Failures on Highway Embankments using Electrical Resistivity Imaging (ERI), Unmanned Aerial Vehicle (UAV), and Finite Element Method (FEM) Numerical Modeling for Forensic Analysis. Transportation Geotechnics 2023;40:100949. https://doi.org/10.1016/j.trgeo.2023.100949.

[40] Mojica A, Pérez T, Toral J, Miranda R, Franceschi P, Calderón C, et al. Shallow electrical resistivity imaging of the Limón fault, Chagres River Watershed, Panama Canal. Journal of Applied Geophysics 2017;138:135-42. https://doi.org/10.1016/j.jappgeo.2017.01.010.

[41] Abidin MHZ, Saad R, Ahmad F, Wijeyesekera DC, Baharuddin MFT. Application of Geophysical Methods in Civil Engineering 2011.

[42] Shevnin V, Mousatov A, Ryjov A, Delgado-Rodriquez O. Estimation of clay content in soil based on resistivity modelling and laboratory measurements. Geophysical Prospecting 2007;55:265-75. https://doi.org/10.1111/j.1365-2478.2007.00599.x.

[43] Brunet P, Clément R, Bouvier C. Monitoring soil water content and deficit using Electrical Resistivity Tomography (ERT) - A case study in the Cevennes area, France. Journal of Hydrology 2010;380:146-53. https://doi.org/10.1016/j.jhydrol.2009.10.032.

[44] Cassiani G, Godio A, Stocco S, Villa A, Deiana R, Frattini P, et al. Monitoring the hydrologic behaviour of a mountain slope via time-lapse electrical resistivity tomography. Near Surface Geophysics 2009;7:475-86. https://doi.org/10.3997/1873-0604.2009013.

[45] Edwards LS. A MODIFIED PSEUDOSECTION FOR RESISTIVITY AND IP. GEOPHYSICS 1977;42:1020–36. https://doi.org/10.1190/1.1440762.

[46] Ducut JD, Alipio M, Go PJ, Concepcion Ii R, Vicerra RR, Bandala A, et al. A Review of Electrical Resistivity Tomography Applications in Underground Imaging and Object Detection. Displays 2022;73:102208. https://doi.org/10.1016/j.displa.2022.102208.

[47] Chambers JE, Gunn DA, Wilkinson PB, Meldrum PI, Haslam E, Holyoake S, et al. 4D electrical resistivity tomography monitoring of soil moisture dynamics in an operational railway embankment. Near Surface Geophysics 2014;12:61-72. https://doi.org/10.3997/1873-0604.2013002.

[48] Li X-J, Marasteanu MO. Using Semi Circular Bending Test to Evaluate Low Temperature Fracture Resistance for Asphalt Concrete. Exp Mech 2010;50:867-76. https://doi.org/10.1007/s11340-009-9303-0.

[49] Dehnad MH, Khodaii A, Moghadas Nejad F. Moisture sensitivity of asphalt mixtures under different load frequencies and temperatures. Construction and Building Materials 2013;48:700-7. https://doi.org/10.1016/j.conbuildmat.2013.07.059.

[50] Aliha MRM, Behbahani H, Fazaeli H, Rezaifar MH. Study of characteristic specification on mixed mode fracture toughness of asphalt mixtures. Construction and Building Materials 2014;54:623-35. https://doi.org/10.1016/j.conbuildmat.2013.12.097.

[51] Aliha MRM, Fazaeli H, Aghajani S, Moghadas Nejad F. Effect of temperature and air void on mixed mode fracture toughness of modified asphalt mixtures. Construction and Building Materials 2015;95:545-55. https://doi.org/10.1016/j.conbuildmat.2015.07.165.

[52] Abuawad IMA, Al-Qadi IL, Trepanier JS. Mitigation of moisture damage in asphalt concrete: Testing techniques and additives/modifiers effectiveness. Construction and Building Materials 2015;84:437-43. https://doi.org/10.1016/j.conbuildmat.2015.03.001.

[53] Lamothe S, Perraton D, Benedetto HD. Degradation of hot mix asphalt samples subjected to freeze-thaw cycles and partially saturated with water or brine. Road Materials and Pavement Design 2017;18:849-64. https://doi.org/10.1080/14680629.2017.1286442.

[54] Ameri M, Vamegh M, Chavoshian Naeni SF, Molayem M. Moisture susceptibility evaluation of asphalt mixtures containing Evonik, Zycotherm and hydrated lime. Construction and Building Materials 2018. https://doi.org/10.1016/j.conbuildmat.2017.12.113.

[55] Fakhri M, Ali Siyadati S, Aliha MRM. Impact of freeze-thaw cycles on low temperature mixed mode I/II cracking properties of water saturated hot mix asphalt: An experimental study. Construction and Building Materials 2020;261:119939. https://doi.org/10.1016/j.conbuildmat.2020.119939.

[56] Fatemi S, Zarei M, Ziaee SA, Shad R, Amir Saadatjoo S, Tabasi E. Low and intermediate temperatures fracture behavior of amorphous poly alpha olefin (APAO)-modified hot mix asphalt subjected to constant and variable temperatures. Construction and Building Materials 2023;364:129840. https://doi.org/10.1016/j.conbuildmat.2022.129840.

[57] Gupta L, Bellary A. Comparative study on The Behavior of Bituminous Concrete Mix and Warm Mix Asphalt Prepared Using Lime and Zycotherm as Additive. Materials Today: Proceedings 2018;5:2074-81. https://doi.org/10.1016/j.matpr.2017.09.203.

[58] NM EN 1097-2. Tests for mechanical and physical properties of aggregates - Part 2: methods for the determination of resistance to fragmentation 2022.

[59] NM EN 1097-1. Tests for mechanical and physical properties of aggregates - Part 1: determination of the resistance to wear (micro-Deval) 2018.

[60] NM EN 933-3. Tests for geometrical properties of aggregates - Part 3: determination of particle shape - Flakiness index 2018.

[61] NM 10.1.169. Aggregates. Determination of surface cleanliness. 2020.

[62] NM EN 933-8. Tests for geometrical properties of aggregates - Part 8: assessment of fines - Sand equivalent test 2022.

[63] NM EN 933-1. Tests for geometrical properties of aggregates - Part 1: determination of particle size distribution - Sieving method 2017.

[64] NF T66-043-2. Bitumen and bituminous binders - Determination of the passive adhesivity of bituminous binders by the water immersion test - Aggregate method - Part 2: unmodified bitumens and modified bitumens 2016.

[65] EN 1097-6. Tests for mechanical and physical properties of aggregates - Part 6: determination of particle density and water absorption 2018.

[66] NM EN 15326. Bitumen and bituminous binders - Measurement of density and specific gravity - Capillary-stoppered Pyknometer method 2017.

[67] NF EN 12697-5. Bituminous mixtures - Test methods - Part 5: determination of the maximum density 2018.

[68] Nsengiyumva G, Kim Y-R, You T. Development of a Semicircular Bend (SCB) Test Method for Performance Testing of Nebraska Asphalt Mixtures 2015.

[69] Zarei M, Salehikalam A, Tabasi E, Naseri A, Worya Khordehbinan M, Negahban M. Pure mode I fracture resistance of hot mix asphalt (HMA) containing nano-SiO2 under freeze-thaw damage (FTD). Construction and Building Materials 2022;351:128757. https://doi.org/10.1016/j.conbuildmat.2022.128757.

[70] Tabasi E, Zarei M, Naseri A, Gashin Hosseini S, Mirahmadi M, Khordehbinan MW. Low temperature cracking behavior of modified asphalt mixture under modes I and III. Theoretical and Applied Fracture Mechanics 2023;128:104150. https://doi.org/10.1016/j.tafmec.2023.104150.

[71] Lu DX, Nguyen NHT, Saleh M, Bui HH. Experimental and numerical investigations of non-standardised semi-circular bending test for asphalt concrete mixtures. International Journal of Pavement Engineering 2021;22:960-72. https://doi.org/10.1080/10298436.2019.1654608.

[72] Lim IL, Johnston IW, Choi SK. Stress intensity factors for semicircular specimens under three-point bending. Engineering Fracture Mechanics 1993;44:363-82. https://doi.org/10.1016/0013-7944(93)90030-V.

[73] EN 12697-44. Bituminous mixtures - Test methods - Part 44: crack propagation by semi-circular bending test 2019.

[74] Sebaaly, PE, Little, . DN, Epps, JA. The Benefits of HYDRATED LIME IN HOT MIX ASPHALT. the National Lime Association; 2006.

[75] Behnia B, Buttlar WG, Reis H. Cooling cycle effects on low temperature cracking characteristics of asphalt concrete mixture. Mater Struct 2014;47:1359-71. https://doi.org/10.1617/s11527-014-0310-y.

[76] Mehrara A, Khodaii A. A review of state of the art on stripping phenomenon in asphalt concrete. Construction and Building Materials 2013;38:423-42. https://doi.org/10.1016/j.conbuildmat.2012.08.033.

[77] Kim KW, Kweon SJ, Doh YS, Park T-S. Fracture toughness of polymer-modified asphalt concrete at low temperatures. Can J Civ Eng 2003;30:406-13. https://doi.org/10.1139/l02-101.

[78] Lesueur D, Petit J, Ritter H-J. The mechanisms of hydrated lime modification of asphalt mixtures: a state-of-the-art review. Road Materials and Pavement Design 2013;14:1-16. https://doi.org/10.1080/14680629.2012.743669.

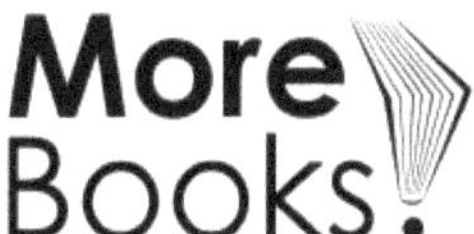

I want morebooks!

Buy your books fast and straightforward online - at one of world's fastest growing online book stores! Environmentally sound due to Print-on-Demand technologies.

Buy your books online at
www.morebooks.shop

Kaufen Sie Ihre Bücher schnell und unkompliziert online – auf einer der am schnellsten wachsenden Buchhandelsplattformen weltweit! Dank Print-On-Demand umwelt- und ressourcenschonend produzi ert.

Bücher schneller online kaufen
www.morebooks.shop

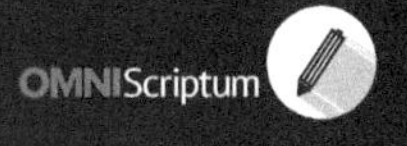

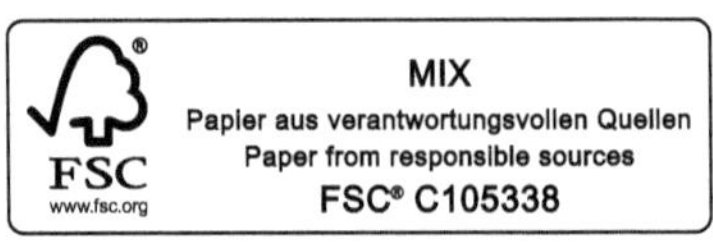

Printed by Books on Demand GmbH, Norderstedt / Germany